Surface Ablation
Techniques for Optimum Results

Surface Ablation
Techniques for Optimum Results

ELLEN E. ANDERSON PENNO, MD, MS, FRCSC
Medical Director
Western Laser Eye Associates
Calgary, Alberta, Canada

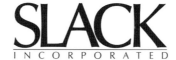

SLACK
INCORPORATED

www.Healio.com/books

ISBN: 978-1-61711-074-0

SLACK Incorporated uses a review process to evaluate submitted material. Prior to publication, educators or clinicians provide important feedback on the content that we publish. We welcome feedback on this work.

Published by: SLACK Incorporated
                   6900 Grove Road
                   Thorofare, NJ 08086 USA
                   Telephone: 856-848-1000
                   Fax: 856-848-6091
                   `www.Healio.com/books

Contact SLACK Incorporated for more information about other books in this field or about the availability of our books from distributors outside the United States.

Library of Congress Cataloging-in-Publication Data

Surface ablation : techniques for optimum results / [edited by] Ellen Anderson Penno, MD.
       p. ; cm.
  Includes bibliographical references and index.
  ISBN 978-1-61711-074-0 (pbk. : alk. paper)
  I. Penno, Ellen E. Anderson, editor of compilation.
  [DNLM: 1. Refractive Surgical Procedures--methods. 2. Cornea--surgery. 3. Corneal Surgery, Laser--methods. 4. Treatment Outcome. WW 340]

  617.7'190598--dc23
                        2012048561

Printed in the United States of America.

Last digit is print number: 10 9 8 7 6 5 4 3 2 1

DEDICATION

For my family, who continue to provide patience, love, and support.

CONTENTS

ACKNOWLEDGMENTS

Writing a book is always a collaboration, as is the practice of medicine. Thank you to all of the contributors for sharing your perspectives on surface ablation topics. Refractive surgery continues to evolve and improve due to the efforts of ophthalmologists who are willing to share their knowledge through meetings, research, journal articles, and books such as this.

All of the staff at SLACK Incorporated, including John Bond, Senior Vice President of Health Care Books and Journals as well as the editors, marketing, and production staff, have been instrumental in bringing this book from a concept to a completed manuscript.

A heartfelt thank you is also due to my mentor Dr. Howard Gimbel, who continues to be an innovator in the field of refractive surgery. As a co-author of previous books published by SLACK Incorporated, Dr. Gimbel and the staff of the Gimbel Eye Centre have been important to the success of these writing projects over the years. As a clinical mentor, Dr. Gimbel has provided valuable insights through his experience and expertise.

Thank you to my staff at Western Laser Eye Associates and, in particular, my office manager Michele Hymas, who have supported my efforts in developing clinical practices and materials, some of which are included in this book.

A thank you is due also to the many patients over the years who have and continue to provide valuable feedback through both outcomes and feedback.

ABOUT THE AUTHOR

Ellen E. Anderson Penno, MD, MS, FRCSC, of Western Laser Eye Associates is an eye surgeon and author who has resided in the Calgary area for more than 10 years. Trained at the Mayo Clinic in Rochester, Minnesota with a refractive fellowship at the Gimbel Eye Centre in Calgary, Alberta, she has been practicing refractive surgery and general ophthalmology since 1996 and has performed thousands of surgeries on a variety of laser types. Dr. Anderson Penno is a Fellow of the Royal College of Physicians in Canada and a Diplomate of the American Board of Ophthalmology.

Writing has always been a part of Dr. Anderson Penno's career. In addition to numerous peer-reviewed articles and book chapters, she co-authored the book *LASIK Complications* with Dr. Howard Gimbel. Additional writing activities include articles for Salem Press and serving as a peer reviewer for the *Journal of Cataract and Refractive Surgery.*

Dr. Anderson Penno lives and works in Calgary, Alberta, Canada and founded Western Laser Eye Associates in 2004.

CONTRIBUTING AUTHORS

David P. Chan, MD (Chapter 11)
Surgical Fellow, Anterior Segment and
    Refractive Surgery
Gimbel Eye Centre
University of Calgary
Calgary, Alberta, Canada

Richard J. Duffey, MD (Chapter 7)
Premier Medical Eye Group
Mobile, Alabama

Daniel S. Durrie, MD (Chapter 4)
Clinical Professor of Ophthalmology
University of Kansas Medical Center
Overland Park, Kansas

Howard V. Gimbel, MD, MPH, FRCSC,
    FACS (Foreword, Chapter 11)
Professor and Chair, Department of
    Ophthalmology
Loma Linda University
Loma Linda, California
Clinical Professor, Department of Surgery
University of Calgary
Calgary, Alberta
Clinical Professor, Department of
    Ophthalmology
University of California
San Francisco, California
Executive Medical Director
Cataract and Refractive Surgeon
Gimbel Eye Centre
Alberta, Canada

Harilaos Ginis, PhD (Chapter 2)
Research Fellow
University of Crete
Department of Medicine
Institute of Vision and Optics
Heraklion, Greece

Maria Kalyvianaki, PhD, MD (Chapter 2)
Institute of Vision and Optics
Medical School, University of Crete
Crete, Greece

Alejandro Lichtinger, MD (Chapter 1)
Cornea, External Ocular Diseases and
    Refractive Surgery Fellow
University of Toronto
Toronto, Ontario, Canada

Ioannis Pallikaris, PhD, MD (Chapter 2)
University of Crete
School of Health Sciences
Crete, Greece

Theodore A. Pasquali, MD (Chapter 4)
Fellow in Cornea and Refractive Surgery
Durrie Vision
Overland Park, Kansas

J. Bradley Randleman, MD (Chapter 8)
Professor of Ophthalmology
Director, Cornea, External Disease, and
    Refractive Surgery
Emory Vision and Emory University
Department of Ophthalmology
Atlanta, Georgia

David S. Rootman, MD, FACS (Chapter 1)
Professor, University of Toronto
Department of Ophthalmology and Vision
    Sciences
Medical Director, Yonge Eglinton Laser Eye
    Centre
Toronto, Ontario, Canada

Rupa D. Shah, MD (Chapter 8)
Assistant Professor of Ophthalmology
Case Western Reserve University
Attending Physician
Metrohealth Medical Center
Cleveland, Ohio

FOREWORD

Corneal refractive surgery has evolved to include a number of techniques and technologies since the introduction of radial keratotomy (RK). Diurnal variations in the refraction of some RK eyes made for a less-than-optimal outcome, especially those with high myopic corrections. Also, higher-order aberrations were not uncommon due to the placement of incisions and variable curvature change from incisions in thinner and thicker parts of the cornea.

The precision of laser corneal refractive surgery compared to the somewhat uncertain outcomes of RK made photorefractive keratectomy (PRK) a welcomed new modality for the correction of myopia with corneal surgery. However, quality of vision was too often compromised with the healing response of haze in moderate to high corrections. Without tracking systems in the early excimer lasers, the irregular surface of the ablated area was the frequent source of haze. When laser in situ keratomileusis (LASIK) was introduced, not only was there an enthusiasm for the quick healing response, but the LASIK flap, by maintaining an intact epithelium and Bowman's membrane, had virtually eliminated the occurrence of postoperative corneal surface haze.

Early LASIK technology had a new set of potential problems, such as possible suction breaks with partial flaps, button-holed flaps, variable flap thickness, flap striae, interface inflammation, and a higher risk of ectasia, than was occurring after PRK.

With the advances in laser technology, such as tracking systems, optional epithelial removal techniques, and medications such as mitomycin C, the risks of corneal surface ablation techniques have been lowered. This excellent book by Dr. Anderson Penno and co-authors elaborates on these and other advances and gives the reader valuable information needed to enhance surface ablation outcomes and to aid the surgeon in choosing from all of the options for corneal refractive surgery. It is comprehensive, well-organized, and timely.

We have learned from the history of corneal refractive surgery and other surgeries, such as cataract surgery, that change is to be expected. We have to be open and ready to adopt changes, which sometimes, as with surface ablation, means going back to previously popular procedures with different techniques and technologies to achieve enhanced results or have fewer risks of complications. An example of this is simultaneous corneal collagen cross-linking at the time of corneal surface ablation or LASIK to hopefully reduce the risk of corneal ectasia and achieve a more stable refractive result in some types of refractive corrections. We need to expect further innovative developments that may take us to new procedures or modifications of current procedures.

Howard V. Gimbel, MD, MPH, FRCSC, FACS
Professor and Chair, Department of Ophthalmology
Loma Linda University
Loma Linda, California
Clinical Professor, Department of Surgery
University of Calgary
Calgary, Alberta
Clinical Professor, Department of Ophthalmology
University of California
San Francisco, California
Executive Medical Director
Cataract and Refractive Surgeon
Gimbel Eye Centre
Alberta, Canada

INTRODUCTION

Surface Ablation: Techniques for Optimum Results is intended for both new refractive surgeons who want to learn about surface ablation and experienced surgeons who may be transitioning back to no-flap treatments.

Following Dr. McDonald's first PRK in the 1980s, excimer laser refractive surgery has continued to grow. Early PRK surgeries were complicated by some issues of haze formation, particularly in high corrections. With the introduction of corneal flaps by Dr. Pallikaris in the 1990s, LASIK became the surgery of choice due to faster recovery, less discomfort following surgery, and a reduction of haze.

As the popularity of LASIK increased, so did the recognition of complications. A number of potential complications can occur with LASIK, and this was the subject of *LASIK Complications,* published by SLACK Incorporated. The most feared complication of LASIK continues to be corneal ectasia. While surface ablation can lead to ectasia, it is much less common.

More recently, improved technology, including wavefront excimer laser capabilities combined with continued concern about risk of corneal ectasia, has led to renewed interest in surface ablation. New techniques including LASEK and epi-LASIK were developed in order to improve on PRK results. Despite improvements in flap-making technology with the femtosecond laser, there continues to be renewed interest in surface ablation. Some surgeons have incorporated surface ablation more often as an option for patients who are felt to be at higher risk for ectasia and others have switched completely to surface ablation. In the coming years, surface ablation will continue to be a growing part of many practices.

Surface Ablation: Techniques for Optimum Results offers a practical approach with clinically useful tips, including patient counselling and postoperative care, that will improve patient satisfaction. Surface ablation does require careful counselling due to the longer recovery. With an efficient pre- and postoperative routine, chair time can be optimized and the patient can benefit from improved safety and excellent results. This up-to-date book will be an excellent resource for refractive surgeons.

After more than 10 years of practice, thousands of flaps, and a book called *LASIK Complications,* I have rediscovered the simplicity and outstanding results of surface ablation. While some patients still seek the quick fix offered with flap-based refractive surgeries, a growing number of patients and surgeons are opting for the safety of surface ablation. As with all refractive surgeries, the preoperative work of proper patient selection and setting appropriate expectations is the key to success. Encouraging patients to take appropriate time off for recovery is essential.

Surface ablation continues to gain popularity even in the face of exciting improvements in flap creation technology with the advent of the femtosecond laser. More and more patients are asking for PRK or other no-flap treatments as a safer alternative. This book outlines ways to optimize results and patient satisfaction with surface ablation techniques.

Ellen E. Anderson Penno, MD, MS, FRCSC

1

Back to the Surface
The Rise and Fall and Rise Again of Surface Ablation

"Sizzle or Steak" was the recent title of an article by Steinert discussing new developments in refractive surgery.[1] Surface ablation is definitely steak. In an environment where patients and surgeons are constantly looking for the next best thing, photorefractive keratectomy (PRK) has persisted for more than a quarter of a century. There have been profound advancements in diagnostic equipment, treatment technology, and medications that have allowed surface ablation to continue over the years as a safe and effective refractive technique.

HISTORY OF SURFACE ABLATION

Surface ablation started with PRK in the 1980s with the development of the excimer laser, which provided an alternative to incisional refractive surgery. Refractive techniques have expanded to include PRK, laser epithelial keratomileusis (LASEK), and epithelial laser in situ keratomileusis (epi-LASIK) (Table 1-1). All surface ablation techniques involve removal of the corneal epithelium followed by excimer laser ablation to the underlying cornea to achieve a refractive correction.

In some cases, a smoothing effect is achieved by ablation of the epithelium or the use of smoothing techniques after epithelial removal as in phototherapeutic keratectomy (PTK). To understand what has allowed surface ablation to remain as a refractive technique for more than 25 years, it helps to look back at prior refractive surgery techniques and why techniques were eventually changed or abandoned (Table 1-2).

Methods of reshaping the corneal surface to correct refractive errors prior to the excimer laser included radial keratotomy (RK) and lamellar keratoplasty. The use of incisions for the treatment of myopia was first attempted by Lans at the end of the 19th century. Throughout the next several decades, surgeons including Sato attempted to refine the technique of using posterior and anterior radial incisions to create corneal flattening. The method was refined to include only anterior incisions and the number of incisions was reduced.

By the 1970s, Fyodorov made RK famous with his assembly line approach to refractive surgery with multiple surgeons operating on multiple patients simultaneously.

"This institute should be called Medical Factory No. 1 for production of people with good eyesight," Fyodorov told the Associated Press in 1985. According to some reports, it was Fyodorov's observation of a young boy with a corneal injury that led to the development of his RK technique.

Anderson Penno EE. *Surface Ablation: Techniques for Optimum Results (pp 1-14).* © 2013 SLACK Incorporated.

TABLE 1-1. SURFACE ABLATION TECHNIQUES

Photorefractive keratectomy—PRK
Phototherapeutic keratectomy—PTK
Laser-assisted subepithelial keratomileusis—LASEK
Epithelial laser in situ keratomileusis—epi-LASIK

TABLE 1-2. REFRACTIVE SURGERY EVOLUTION

TECHNIQUE	
RK	Incisional surgery made popular by Fyodorov in the 1970s; diurnal fluctuations, progressive hyperopia
PRK	First-generation excimer laser surgery introduced by McDonald and Seiler in the 1980s; corneal haze (less common today), pain and recovery time, ectasia less common with PRK
LASIK	Introduced by Dr. Pallikaris and other surgeons around the world in the 1990s; combined excimer laser with a lamellar flap; ectasia, flap complications
Intra-LASIK	Introduced in 2000; uses the femtosecond laser to create a corneal flap; ectasia; flap complications; photophobia
LASEK	An attempt to eliminate risks associated with haze, pain, recovery time with a stromal flap while maintaining benefits of rapid healing by creating an epithelial flap
Epi-LASIK	Modification of LASEK; uses automated device to create epithelial flap; discarding the flap may speed healing haze, pain, recovery time
SBK	Sub-Bowman's keratomileusis is a modification of LASIK with an ultrathin flap; flap complications, ectasia risk theoretically lower with a thinner flap

He noted that after having lost a part of the corneal surface, the boy's myopia was reduced. Fyodorov's precedent of high-volume surgery set the stage for the high-volume refractive surgeons to follow.

The technique widely used in the United States during this decade used a diamond knife to make radial incisions that resulted in a flattening effect, thereby correcting myopia. Complication rates were low but included microperforations, macroperforations requiring suturing, loss of best-corrected acuity, irregular astigmatism, glare, fluctuating vision, and, more rarely, neovascularization and keratitis.

While the results of RK were still somewhat variable, the overall success of the procedure made it an attractive alternative to many surgeons and patients for the treatment of myopia around the world. In the late 1970s, Bores performed the first RK in the United States. RK had to achieve a high level of safety because it was an elective procedure. Candidates for RK could obtain good vision with glasses or contact lenses and during this period of time, it was not widely accepted that it would be appropriate to take the risk of corneal surgery simply to reduce dependence on corrective lenses.

There were still many ophthalmologists in the 1980s who were opposed to the concept of performing elective surgery within the visual axis of a healthy eye. Taking a risk with eyes that could correct well with glasses or contact lenses was considered to be reckless by some surgeons during

TABLE 1-3. INTRODUCTION OF OPHTHALMIC LASERS

1960.......Helium neon laser developed at Bell Laboratories

1963.......Ruby laser for retinal photocoagulation

1963.......First diode pumper solid-state laser developed at the Massachussets Institute of Technology

1968.......Argon laser for retinal photocoagulation

1980.......Nd:YAG for posterior capsulotomy

1987.......Erbium YAG used for photoablation of ocular tissue

1995.......Excimer laser FDA approved for PRK

2000.......Femtosecond laser for corneal flap creation

the era of refractive surgery. It was a paradigm shift that would gain momentum over the next decade.

By 1981, the National Eye Institute launched the Prospective Evaluation of Radial Keratotomy (PERK) study. In 1994, the 10-year results were released, which concluded that 250,000 RK surgeries were being performed each year in the United States and that RK was a "reasonably safe" method of correcting myopia.[2] The report also included mention of progressive hyperopic shifts post-RK. Reports of diurnal fluctuations following RK appeared in the published literature.[3,4]

Simultaneous to the refinements of RK for the treatment of myopia, Barraquer was working on lamellar refractive surgery. Keratophakia, keratomileusis, and epikeratoplasty were techniques that involved reshaping corneal discs to correct refractive errors. From 1949 with his first paper on lamellar refractive keratoplasty through the 1980s, Barraquer and other surgeons worked to improve techniques of lamellar keratoplasty.[5] Barraquer is credited with inventing the first microkeratome. These lamellar refractive surgery techniques did not achieve the widespread popularity of RK, but did form the basis for what was to become the most popular technique by the late 1990s—laser-assisted in situ keratomileusis (LASIK).

During the same time period, lasers were developed for a wide variety of applications. Lasers began to be used for the treatment of retinal disorders in the 1960s and 1970s (Table 1-3). The initial lasers created a photocoagulation effect similar to cautery. Later lasers generated photodisruption within tissues. Laser use has expanded to include applications in the treatment of glaucoma and posterior capsular fibrosis, in addition to a number of retinal conditions.

Excimer lasers create photoablation of tissue, which causes an effect like evaporation such that the tissue bonds are broken and the material is aerosolized without thermal damage to the underlying tissue (Figure 1-1). The excimer laser was developed originally for etching computer chips but in 1981, Srinivasan and his colleagues discovered that the excimer laser could precisely cut organic material.

According to some reports, Srinivasan brought his leftover Thanksgiving turkey to the laboratory to experiment with the excimer laser, which led him to the discovery that the excimer laser could precisely remove organic tissue without burning or destroying the underlying tissue. The timing of this discovery coincided with the increased popularity of RK.

Investigators later worked with Trokel, who used the excimer to create corneal incisions. Numerous investigators subsequently worked to refine the use of the excimer laser for corneal refractive surgery through animal studies and human blind eye studies resulting in the technique of central ablation rather than radial incisions. Seiler and McDonald are credited with the first surface ablation surgeries on sighted eyes in the 1980s.[6,7] By 1997, PRK became the preferred method for treating low myopia.

Figure 1-1. Excimer laser technology continues to evolve and now includes the ability to perform wavefront-guided ablation profiles. (Photograph by Amanda Sneddon.)

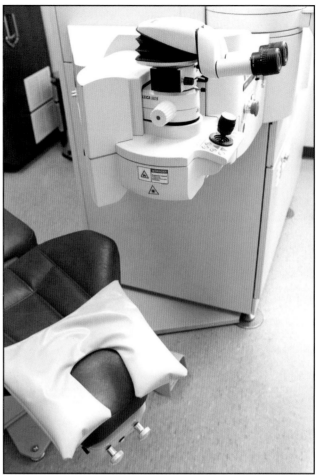

LASIK Revolution

In the early 1990s, there were reports of haze and night vision disturbances following PRK. Pallikaris, Buratto, and others began to use the prior lamellar techniques in combination with excimer laser ablation to create LASIK.[8] LASIK quickly became the refractive procedure of choice for high myopia due to the reduced risk of haze and rapid recovery of vision as compared to PRK. By 1998, LASIK was the procedure of choice for all levels of myopia. By 2003, RK was no longer a procedure of choice for US surgeons even for low myopia.

Excimer laser ablation was proving to be safe enough to consider simultaneous bilateral surgery. This was another paradigm shift in the practice of corneal refractive surgery. The practice of bilateral excimer laser ablation has become the standard for most refractive surgeons with few exceptions. This approach offers the convenience of fewer appointments and quicker recovery for refractive surgery patients.

Back to the Surface

As the volume of LASIK surgeries increased, reports of complications including ectasia increased. During the late 1990s, there were many articles, books, and presentations at meetings

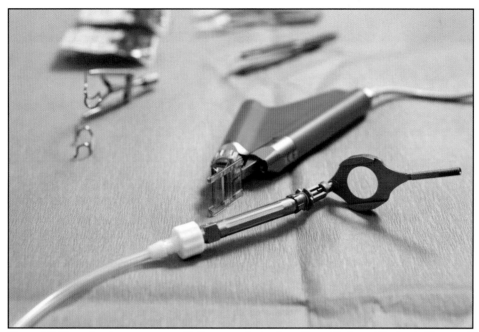

Figure 1-2. The epikeratome uses an oscillating separator to cleave the epithelium at the level of Bowman's membrane. The resulting sheet of epithelium can be repositioned for LASEK (also called epi-LASIK) or removed for flap-off epi-LASIK. (Photograph by Amanda Sneddon.)

about LASIK complications and how to avoid them. While the complication rate was low, there were a number of possible risks, including flap complications, shifted flaps, epithelial ingrowth, diffuse lamellar keratitis, and the most feared complication—ectasia. Reports of corneal ectasia peaked in 2001 but it remains a concern of refractive surgeons due to the difficulty in accurately predicting which corneas are at risk and the difficulty in treating resulting corneal instability.

Surgeons worked to find a technique that avoided the potential flap complications of LASIK but that offered the more rapid recovery that LASIK provided. The Amoils brush, a rotating brush for the removal of epithelium for PRK, was developed in the mid-1990s. Through the early years of this century, McDonald, Pallikaris, Camellin, and many others worked to perfect the new technique of laser-assisted subepithelial keratomileusis (LASEK), which in theory would create a viable epithelial flap that could be reflected back into place following laser ablation.[9] During the past several years, there has been a lot of discussion on whether to save the epithelium, and many surgeons elect to discard the flap.

Pallikaris is credited with the invention of the epikeratome, which uses a blunt oscillating separator to push away the epithelium using Bowman's membrane to guide the separator smoothly along the epithelial junction (Figure 1-2). This technique has been called epi-LASIK. Corneas with scarring or irregularities involving Bowman's membrane would not be suited for epi-LASIK. The rationale behind epi-LASIK is to avoid the use of dilute alcohol, which may devitalize the epithelial flap cells.

Technological Advancements

Since the excimer laser was introduced, there have been impressive advancements in the technology for preoperative assessment, laser ablation, and surgical technology. On the diagnostic side, corneal mapping has advanced to include keratoconus detection software in order to more

TABLE 1-4. ADVANCES IN REFRACTIVE SURGERY DIAGNOSTICS

Keratoconus detection software	Available on topographers to aid in keratoconus screening
Aberrometer	Measurement of higher-order aberrations Used in wavefront treatments and diagnostics
Ocular response analyzer	Measurement of corneal hysteresis May be useful for risk assessment
Optical coherence tomography	Used for corneal and posterior segment imaging

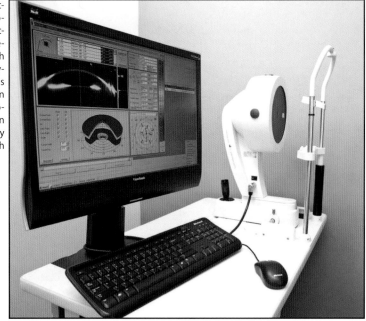

Figure 1-3. Advances in refractive surgery diagnostic equipment include the use of a rotating Scheimpflug camera to create a detailed corneal map, which includes topographic and pachymetric information. Keratoconus detection software has been added to this and other topographic units to aid surgeons in the detection of corneas that may be at risk for ectasia. (Photograph by Amanda Sneddon.)

accurately identify corneas at higher risk for corneal ectasia (Table 1-4). Initially, topography was performed using Placido ring technology, which was limited to the surface topography.

Developments in mapping included the scanning-slit and the rotating Scheimpflug camera that can give additional information about corneal thickness, posterior corneal curvature, and anterior chamber depth (Figure 1-3). Wavefront mapping has allowed for the measurement of higher-order aberrations and for wavefront ablation and wavefront-guided ablation. Surgical advancements in surface ablation have included the development of the epikeratome. Improvements in excimer lasers include improved tracking, iris registration, smoother ablation profiles, variable repetition rates, and wavefront-optimized and wavefront-guided ablations.

The femtosecond laser is the latest laser to be put to use for ophthalmic surgery. The femtosecond laser is an ultra-fast laser that creates a photochemistry effect that is now used to create a corneal flap in intra-LASIK. Microkeratomes have also been developed that produce a thinner corneal flap for LASIK. This technique is called sub-Bowman's keratomileusis. It is not clear from the literature at this time if there is a true reduction in the rate of ectasia as compared to LASIK with sub-Bowman's flaps.

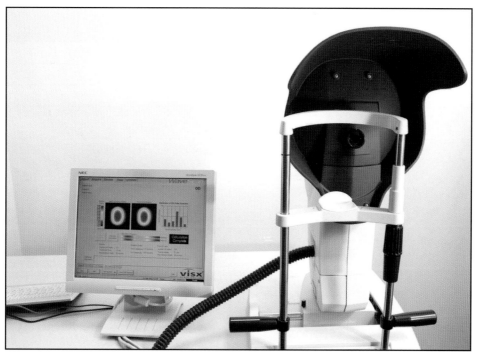

Figure 1-4. Wavefront aberrations can be measured, and the measurements can be used to generate a customized wavefront ablation profile that will treat higher-order aberrations in addition to sphere and cylinder refractive errors. (WaveScan system, Abbott Medical Optics Inc; photograph by Amanda Sneddon.)

Developments in medications since the introduction of the excimer laser include mitomycin C, which is now used routinely for surface ablation in order to reduce the incidence of haze in higher corrections. A number of topical nonsteroidal anti-inflammatory medications are now available including ketorolac and diclofenac. Topical cyclosporine A for treatment of dry eye has become commonplace. Topical steroid choices now include rimexolone and, more recently, difluprednate. Difluprednate is an emulsion that has higher potency and more consistent delivery than other topical steroid suspensions. Fourth-generation fluoroquinolones are used routinely for prophylactic postoperative coverage.

Corneal cross-linking is one of the newer developments at this time. This procedure uses a photosensitive solution of riboflavin (vitamin B_2), which is applied to the corneal surface followed by exposure to UV light. This process creates additional bonds or cross-links between the collagen fibers within corneal stroma. These additional bonds add strength to the cornea. Cross-linking is a technique that has been used to treat post-LASIK ectasia and keratoconus in combination with surface ablation. Some surgeons are incorporating cross-linking as a preventative technique for corneal refractive surgery as discussed in Chapter 11.

The ability to apply wavefront technology to excimer laser ablation represents another leap forward (Figure 1-4). This is another factor that has boosted interest in surface ablation, as there are some surgeons who feel the benefit of correcting higher-order aberrations is increased if it is not masked by a corneal flap of any type. There will likely continue to be lively debate about this in the coming years.

Other refractive techniques that have been developed since the advent of PRK include conductive keratoplasty and corneal ring segments. These techniques have not gained the same popularity as the excimer laser surgeries. Corneal ring segments are used in the treatment of keratoconus and have been combined with corneal cross-linking with good results.

TABLE 1-5. REFRACTIVE SURGERY TRENDS*			
YEAR	SURFACE ABLATION	LASIK	TOTAL
2005	127,000 (11.9%)	939,000 (88.1%)	1,066,000
2010	280,000 (29.2%)	680,000 (70.8%)	960,000
*Figures reported in *Ophthalmology Times*, May 15, 2011 "Data Track Refractive Surgery" from the 2010 ISRS member survey by Dr. Duffey and Dr. Leaming.			

While flap-based techniques including intra-LASIK and LASIK remain the predominant refractive surgery technique, surface ablation has become more popular over the past several years (Table 1-5). Surface ablation includes PRK, LASEK, and epi-LASIK. Some surgeons reserve surface ablation for thin corneas or suspicious corneal mapping. Others have switched completely to surface ablation for all patients.

SAFETY

It is a tribute to the success of RK and subsequent excimer laser refractive surgery that today's patients demand outstanding results and low risks. The expectation for successful outcomes has put pressure on surgeons to continue to provide the latest and best refractive care available. Surface ablation techniques have continued to deliver excellent results with a low complication rate over a number of decades.

A benchmark for safety of refractive surgery has been a comparison to the risk of contact lens wear. There have been studies that indicate that the risk of corneal refractive surgery is similar to the risk of wearing contact lenses.[10] Another way to describe this is that refractive surgery may be as safe as contact lens wear. There are several factors to consider in order to determine if this is true, including contact lens wear habits, such as overwear, lens type, and unusual factors, such as possible solution contaminants, which may increase the risk of *Acanthamoeba* or other corneal infections.

Many patients will also be motivated to consider refractive surgery due to cost. The ongoing cost of glasses or contact lenses over a number of years may exceed the cost of refractive surgery. Cost can also influence the type of refractive surgery a patient may choose. Surgeons and surgery centers will be influenced by cost in terms of what they may choose to offer. Surface ablation has a favorable cost versus benefit profile. In its simplest form, PRK with dilute alcohol provides excellent results with a lower cost than microkeratome or femtosecond laser treatments.

FUTURE OF SURFACE ABLATION

Advances in surface ablation during the past 2 decades have been outstanding. At the present time, the majority of studies indicate that surface ablation and techniques using corneal flaps are equal in efficacy and safety.[11] As discussed in more detail in Chapter 11, surface ablation is a versatile technique that is becoming a staple in practices that include corneal inlays, refractive lensectomy, and phakic intraocular lenses. Surface ablation is also being used in combination with cross-linking in normal cases and in keratoconus treatment.

The next decades will most likely include developments in technology, medication, and techniques that will increase safety, improve quality of vision, decrease postoperative pain, and speed recovery of surface ablation. It is likely that surface ablation will continue to gain popularity over

THE ROLE OF SURFACE ABLATION IN THE TREATMENT OF KERATOCONUS

Alejandro Lichtinger, MD and David S. Rootman, MD, FACS

Keratoconus is a disease of corneal collagen characterized by progressive corneal thinning and irregular steepening of the cornea with a loss of best-corrected visual acuity (BCVA). In the past, the techniques available to improve vision in patients with keratoconus were limited to spectacles, contact lenses, and, in the most severe cases, lamellar or penetrating keratoplasty. In the past 10 years, we have witnessed the introduction of new technologies that, alone or when combined, allow for the reshaping and strengthening of the cornea, resulting in improved BCVA and uncorrected visual acuity (UCVA), while stabilizing the cornea to prevent progression or worsening of the ectatic process. These technologies include topography-guided PRK, Intacs (Addition Technology, Sunnyvale, California), and other intra-corneal ring segments for keratoconus and corneal collagen cross-linking (CXL), all of which have received a Conformité Européenne (CE) mark for clinical use in Europe (2003, 2003, and 2006, respectively).

Excimer laser correction of the refractive error in keratoconus has been previously attempted with variable success concerning predictability and stability.[1-8] LASIK is considered to be contraindicated in keratoconus. More than 60 cases of postoperative keratectasia have been reported,[9] while the number of iatrogenic keratectasia cases reported after surface ablation are limited.[8,10-16]

From the different surface ablation profiles, a wavefront-guided ablation has the advantage that it can treat the whole visual system, including lenticular optical errors and optical errors of the posterior cornea.[3] However, wavefront-guided analysis frequently does not yield reliable results in highly aberrant eyes,[17] as is the case in keratoconus. Topography-guided PRK has the advantage that it flattens not only some of the cone peak but also an arcuate, broader area of cornea away from the cone; this ablation pattern resembles in part a hyperopic treatment and thus will cause some amount of steepening, or elevation, adjacent to the cone (usually in the flatter, superior area), effectively normalizing the cornea.[18] Another advantage of a topography-guided approach is that it reduces the amount of tissue removed compared with a wavefront-guided ablation from the cone apex, which corresponds to the thinnest part of the cornea.[19]

Koller and colleagues[3] reported on the use of topography-guided surface ablation for forme fruste keratoconus in a prospective study of 11 eyes followed for 1 year after the surgery, showing stable or improved BCVA and UCVA and a significant reduction of the refractive error. Similarly, Cennamo and colleagues[9] published a prospective study in which 25 keratoconic eyes showed clinical improvement and no progression 2 years after topography-guided surface ablation. Although we do not support performing surface ablation without the stabilizing effect of CXL even in eyes with the forme fruste type of the disease, these studies show that topography-guided ablation can improve the optical performance of eyes with keratoconus. Furthermore, a study conducted in rabbits[20] suggested that keratoconus stabilization after surface excimer laser ablation could result from the deposit of newly synthesized type I, type III, and type IV collagen; cellular fibronectin; tenascin; and laminin in the extracellular matrix of the anterior corneal stroma.[9] The lack of ectasia progression seen after topography-guided surface ablation coupled with the improved optical performance seen in some studies makes it a reasonable complement to CXL to both strengthen and reshape the cornea in keratoconus.

Although both Intacs and topography-guided surface ablation are helpful in improving UCVA, BCVA, and contact lens tolerance to a certain degree, they do not address the progressive nature of the disease. In recent years, laboratory studies have suggested that by increasing the collagen cross-linking of the corneal stroma, we are able to increase the stiffness of the cornea with attendant stabilization of the normally progressive disease in keratoconus.[21-24] These findings have been corroborated by clinical studies in which CXL has demonstrated the potential for retarding the progression of keratoconus and ectasia after LASIK.[25-28]

CXL stiffens the corneal stroma and halts the ectatic process but it does not directly address the patient's refractive error. CXL causes a limited spherocylindrical change that ranges from a slight steepening to approximately 2.0 D of flattening.[8] Thus, combining CXL to halt the disease and surface ablation with or without Intacs to improve the visual optics may improve visual function while eliminating or postponing the need for corneal transplantation.

Kanellopoulos and Binder were the first to describe the combined use of CXL and topography-guided PRK.[21] In this first case report, the topography-guided PRK was performed 12 months after the CXL procedure. Eighteen months after the PRK procedure, the patient's UCVA and BCVA had improved from 20/100 and 20/50 at baseline (before CXL) to 20/20 and 20/15, while the other untreated eye continued to progress during the same period. Since then, the combined treatment has evolved into a same-day procedure in which the surface ablation is performed before the CXL. The effectiveness of this same-day procedure has been confirmed in multiple reports with follow-ups as long as 2 to 5 years.[29-31]

The main advantages of this approach include the following[30,32]:

- Minimize the potential superficial stroma scarring resulting from the PRK. The patient avoids 2 de-epithelializations, thus reducing the risk of haze. The risk might also be reduced with this approach due to the temporary keratocyte loss during the first months after CXL.[33,34]

- Laser ablation after CXL can cause a reduction in strength in the ablation area by ablating the superficial part of the CXL-treated cornea. Therefore, the goal of performing the ablation before the CXL—to strengthen the stroma at a uniform depth after removal of tissue—has been accomplished.

- Minimize time away from work. Kanellopoulos reported on the comparison of sequential versus same-day simultaneous CXL and topography-guided PRK.[32] In this study, the same-day procedure group performed superiorly with regards to best spectacle-corrected visual acuity, spherical equivalent reduction, mean K reduction, and corneal haze score. In addition to the previously mentioned advantages of the same-day procedure, the author hypothesized that the superiority might be related to "enhanced" CXL due to better penetration of the riboflavin solution through ablated stroma or the absence of Bowman's layer and that cross-linking the more "normal" corneal shape in the laser pretreated eyes makes them more "resistant" to factors affecting progression.

The combination of topography-guided transepithelial PRK (treatment limited to 70% of the cylinder and up to 70% of the spherical component so as not to remove more than 50 μm) with CXL has been popularized as the Athens protocol.[29,35,36]

Another approach was suggested by Chan and colleagues[37] who reported the use of Intacs followed by CXL in a retrospective comparative case series, demonstrating that eyes that had an inferior Intacs SK followed by CXL had a significantly greater reduction in cylinder and steep and average keratometry compared to eyes with Intacs implantation alone. Since then, other studies have corroborated the additive effect of CXL after Intacs implantation.[38-40]

We have recently reported our results using Intacs followed by same-day PRK and CXL.[41] Once the keratometry readings, UCVA, and BCVA had been stable for at least 6 months, our results showed statistically significant improvements in UCVA, BCVA, manifest refractive spherical equivalent, keratometry readings, and total aberrations. The rationale for this protocol was that the use of Intacs would induce corneal flattening and reduce keratometric astigmatism, allowing controlled PRK treatment to be performed with minimal tissue ablation followed by CXL to stiffen the cornea and halt progression of the ectatic process. The aim of the PRK treatment was to treat part of the refractive error and regularize the cornea rather than fully correct the ametropia.

Another approach we are currently using for cases of keratoconus is to perform same-day single-segment Intacs SK, transepithelial PTK, and CXL in the following sequence:

1. Femtosecond laser (IntraLase FS, Abbott Medical Optics, Abbott Park, Illinois) channel creation for the Intacs at a depth of 400 μm.

2. Trans-epithelial PTK to a depth of 50 μm (VISX Star S4, Abbott Medical Optics, Abbott Park, Illinois). This will usually remove a small amount of the steepest part of the cornea because the epithelium is usually thinnest over the cone. Thus, the epithelium over the cone is removed first followed by limited removal of the steepest part of the cone.

3. Removal of the remaining central 9 mm of corneal epithelium by application of 50% ethanol for 6 seconds using a trephine-guided alcohol chamber (Duckworth and Kent Ltd, Hertfordshire, United Kingdom). A mini-beaver blade is used to mechanically remove the epithelium.

4. Single Intacs SK 450 segment implanted inferiorly.

5. CXL performed by administering 0.1% riboflavin solution (Haber's Pharmacy, Toronto, Canada) every 2 minutes for 30 minutes. Ultraviolet A light (365 nm) is projected onto the cornea with a 12.0-mW/cm^2 surface radiance for 10 minutes (UV-X 2000, IROC, Zurich, Switzerland) while the riboflavin solution is continually applied every 2 minutes.

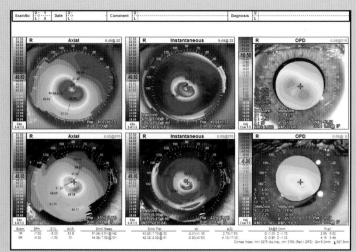

Figure 1A-1. Comparative topography OD.

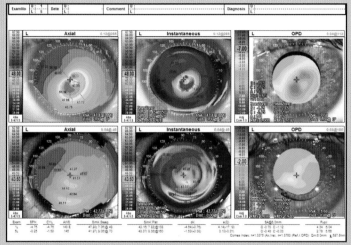

Figure 1A-2. Comparative topography OS.

The following is an example of this latest approach: A 20-year-old woman with progressive keratoconus was referred to us 2 years after CXL elsewhere. On first examination, her UCVA was 20/400 in her right eye, or oculus dexter (OD) and 20/250 in her left eye, or oculus sinister (OS), BCVA was 20/60[+1] with a manifest refraction (MR) of -5.0/-4.25@044 OD and 20/30 with a MR of +2.50/-6.0@111 OS. Keratometry readings were 51.75/43.75 OD and 47.75/42.25 OS.

We implanted a single 0.45-mm Intacs SK inferiorly, followed by transepithelial PTK and CXL in both eyes. A year after the procedure, her UCVA improved to 20/50 OD and 20/25 OS, while her BCVA improved to 20/30[-2] with a MR of -5.00/-2.75@061 OD and 20/20-2 with a MR of +0.50/-1.50@145 OS. Her keratometry readings at last follow-up were 45.00/42.00 OD and 41.75/40.25 OS (a comparative topographic map from preoperative parameters to last follow-up can be seen in Figure 1A-1 for OD and Figure 1A-2 for OS).

Surface ablation in keratoconus has proven helpful in reducing the refractive error and improving the optical quality of the eye, but the long-term progressive instability without the stabilizing effect of CXL makes this therapy controversial at best.[29] CXL has been investigated extensively and has been shown clinically to arrest the progression of keratoconic or post-LASIK ectasia. With its minimal cost, simplicity, and proven positive clinical outcome, CXL can be regarded as a useful approach to reduce the number of penetrating keratoplasties[27] performed and as a revolutionary treatment in the management of keratoconus.

Topography-guided surface ablation combined with CXL is one modality for these very irregular corneas. Our approach has been to combine Intacs with either standard PRK (if done months after the Intacs) or transepithelial PTK (same-day procedure) followed by CXL. Topography-guided PRK might not be as beneficial when placing Intacs segments during the same procedure due to the marked corneal curvature and optical changes that occur with Intacs implantation. The advantage of our approach is that less tissue is removed from an already thin cornea, and reshaping is achieved through an additive approach (Intacs).

Many questions remain unanswered regarding the ideal protocol for the management of keratoconus, such as how much ectasia or type of ectasia we can predictably correct, which treatments are best to combine, the ideal ablation profile and amount of sphere and cylinder to treat, as well as modifications to the CXL procedure currently under study, such as different riboflavin concentrations and solutions, different light sources and irradiance, and epithelium-on treatments among others. Furthermore, the long-term effect of these treatments, while they seem to be stable, needs to be followed for longer periods.

Summary

We can say that surface ablation in its different modalities when combined with CXL has the potential for creating a stable optical improvement of these very irregular corneas, providing not only an arrest of the progression of the keratoconus, but an improvement in visual acuity and quality.

References

1. Fagerholm P, Fitzsimmons T, Ohman L, Orndahl M. Nebulae at keratoconus—the result after excimer laser removal. *Acta Ophthalmol (Copenh).* 1993;71(6):830-832.
2. Alpins N, Stamatelatos G. Customized photoastigmatic refractive keratectomy using combined topographic and refractive data for myopia and astigmatism in eyes with forme fruste and mild keratoconus. *J Cataract Refract Surg.* 2007;33(4):591-602.
3. Koller T, Iseli HP, Donitzky C, et al. Topography-guided surface ablation for forme fruste keratoconus. *Ophthalmology.* 2006;113(12):2198-2202.
4. Kasparova EA, Kasparov AA. Six-year experience with excimer laser surgery for primary keratoconus in Russia. *J Refract Surg.* 2003;19(2 suppl):S250-S254.
5. Appiotti A, Gualdi M. Treatment of keratoconus with laser in situ keratomileusis, photorefractive keratectomy, and radial keratotomy. *J Refract Surg.* 1999;15(2 suppl):S240-S242.
6. Kremer I, Shochot Y, Kaplan A, Blumenthal M. Three year results of photoastigmatic refractive keratectomy for mild and atypical keratoconus. *J Cataract Refract Surg.* 1998;24(12):1581-1588.
7. Reznik J, Salz JJ, Klimava A. Development of unilateral corneal ectasia after PRK with ipsilateral preoperative forme fruste keratoconus. *J Refract Surg.* 2008;24(8):843-847.
8. Randleman JB, Caster AI, Banning CS, Stulting RD. Corneal ectasia after photorefractive keratectomy. *J Cataract Refract Surg.* 2006;32(8):1395-1398.
9. Cennamo G, Intravaja A, Boccuzzi D, Marotta G. Treatment of keratoconus by topography-guided customized photorefractive keratectomy: two-year follow-up study. *J Refract Surg.* 2008;24(2):145-149.
10. Miyata K, Takahashi T, Tomidokoro A, et al. Iatrogenic keratectasia after phototherapeutic keratectomy. *Br J Ophthalmol.* 2001;85(2):247-248.
11. Malecaze F, Coullet J, Calvas P, et al. Corneal ectasia after photorefractive keratectomy for low myopia. *Ophthalmology.* 2006;113(5):742-746.
12. Chiou AG, Bovet J, de Courten C. Management of corneal ectasia and cataract following photorefractive keratectomy. *J Cataract Refract Surg.* 2006;32(4):679-680.
13. Kim H, Choi JS, Joo CK. Corneal ectasia after PRK: clinicopathologic case report. *Cornea.* 2006;25(7):845-848.
14. Leccisotti A. Corneal ectasia after photorefractive keratectomy. *Graefes Arch Clin Exp Ophthalmol.* 2007;245(6):869-875.
15. Amoils P. Corneal ectasia after photorefractive keratectomy. *J Cataract Refract Surg.* 2007;33(6):941-942.
16. Navas A, Ariza E, Haber A, et al. Bilateral keratectasia after photorefractive keratectomy. *J Refract Surg.* 2007;23(9):941-943.
17. Wang L, Wang N, Koch DD. Evaluation of refractive error measurements of the Wavescan Wavefront system and the Tracey Wavefront aberrometer. *J Cataract Refract Surg.* 2003;29(5):970-979.

18. Kanellopoulos AJ. Managing highly distorted corneas with topography-guided Tretament. ISRS/AAO 2007 Subspecialty Day/Refractive Surgery Syllabus 2007; San Francisco, California: American Academy of Ophthalmology.

19. Kanellopoulos AJ, Pe LH. Wavefront-guided enhancements using the wavelight excimer laser in symptomatic eyes previously treated with LASIK. *J Refract Surg.* 2006;22(4):345-349.

20. Qi H, Chen Y, Zhu X. [Studies on the change of extracellular matrix in the corneal tissue after photorefractive keratectomy in rabbits]. *Zhonghua Yan Ke Za Zhi.* 2001;37(2):87-89.

21. Kanellopoulos AJ, Binder PS. Collagen cross-linking (CCL) with sequential topography-guided PRK: a temporizing alternative for keratoconus to penetrating keratoplasty. *Cornea.* 2007;26(7):891-895.

22. Wollensak G, Spoerl E, Seiler T. Riboflavin/ultraviolet-a-induced collagen crosslinking for the treatment of keratoconus. *Am J Ophthalmol.* 2003;135(5):620-627.

23. Spoerl E, Huhle M, Seiler T. Induction of cross-links in corneal tissue. *Exp Eye Res.* 1998;66(1):97-103.

24. Wollensak G, Spoerl E, Seiler T. Stress-strain measurements of human and porcine corneas after riboflavin-ultraviolet-A-induced cross-linking. *J Cataract Refract Surg.* 2003;29(9):1780-1785.

25. Hafezi F, Kanellopoulos J, Wiltfang R, Seiler T. Corneal collagen crosslinking with riboflavin and ultraviolet A to treat induced keratectasia after laser in situ keratomileusis. *J Cataract Refract Surg.* 2007;33(12):2035-2040.

26. Goldich Y, Marcovich AL, Barkana Y, et al. Clinical and corneal biomechanical changes after collagen cross-linking with riboflavin and UV irradiation in patients with progressive keratoconus: results after 2 years of follow-up. *Cornea.* 2012;31(6):609-614.

27. Hovakimyan M, Guthoff RF, Stachs O. Collagen cross-linking: current status and future directions. *J Ophthalmol.* 2012;2012:406850.

28. Wollensak G. Crosslinking treatment of progressive keratoconus: new hope. *Curr Opin Ophthalmol.* 2006;17(4):356-360.

29. Krueger RR, Kanellopoulos AJ. Stability of simultaneous topography-guided photorefractive keratectomy and riboflavin/UVA cross-linking for progressive keratoconus: case reports. *J Refract Surg.* 2010;26(10):S827-832.

30. Stojanovic A, Zhang J, Chen X, et al. Topography-guided transepithelial surface ablation followed by corneal collagen cross-linking performed in a single combined procedure for the treatment of keratoconus and pellucid marginal degeneration. *J Refract Surg.* 2010;26(2):145-152.

31. Labiris G, Giarmoukakis A, Sideroudi H, et al. Impact of keratoconus, cross-linking and cross-linking combined with photorefractive keratectomy on self-reported quality of life. *Cornea.* 2012;31(7):734-739

32. Kanellopoulos AJ. Comparison of sequential vs same-day simultaneous collagen cross-linking and topography-guided PRK for treatment of keratoconus. *J Refract Surg.* 2009;25(9):S812-818.

33. Wollensak G, Spoerl E, Reber F, Seiler T. Keratocyte cytotoxicity of riboflavin/UVA-treatment in vitro. *Eye (Lond).* 2004;18(7):718-722.

34. Mazzotta C, Balestrazzi A, Traversi C, et al. Treatment of progressive keratoconus by riboflavin-UVA-induced cross-linking of corneal collagen: ultrastructural analysis by Heidelberg Retinal Tomograph II in vivo confocal microscopy in humans. *Cornea.* 2007;26(4):390-397.

35. Kanellopoulos AJ. The management of cornea blindness from severe corneal scarring, with the Athens Protocol (transepithelial topography-guided PRK therapeutic remodeling, combined with same-day, collagen cross-linking). *Clin Ophthalmol.* 2012;6:87-90.

36. Kanellopoulos AJ, Binder PS. Management of corneal ectasia after LASIK with combined, same-day, topography-guided partial transepithelial PRK and collagen cross-linking: the athens protocol. *J Refract Surg.* 2011;27(5):323-331.

37. Chan CC, Sharma M, Wachler BS. Effect of inferior-segment Intacs with and without C3-R on keratoconus. *J Cataract Refract Surg.* 2007;33(1):75-80.

38. Kamburoglu G, Ertan A. Intacs implantation with sequential collagen cross-linking treatment in postoperative LASIK ectasia. *J Refract Surg.* 2008;24(7):S726-729.

39. Ertan A, Karacal H, Kamburoglu G. Refractive and topographic results of transepithelial cross-linking treatment in eyes with intacs. *Cornea.* 2009;28(7):719-723.

40. Kilic A, Kamburoglu G, Akinci A. Riboflavin injection into the corneal channel for combined collagen crosslinking and intrastromal corneal ring segment implantation. *J Cataract Refract Surg.* 2012;38(5):878-883.

41. Iovieno A, Legare ME, Rootman DB, et al. Intracorneal ring segments implantation followed by same-day photorefractive keratectomy and corneal collagen cross-linking in keratoconus. *J Refract Surg.* 2011;27(12):915-918.

the next years as a refractive technique and in combination with other methods to treat corneal conditions, such as keratoconus. If the speed of vision recovery could be improved, it may be possible that surface ablation could eventually replace LASIK for primary excimer refractive surgery.

REFERENCES

1. Steinert R. Femto future: sizzle or steak. *Ophthalmology*. 2010;119(5):889-890.
2. Waring GO, Lynn MJ, McDonnell PJ. Results of the prospective evaluation of radial keratotomy (PERK) study 10 years after surgery. *Arch Ophthalmol*. 1994;112(10):1298-1308.
3. Kemp JR, Martinez CE, Klyce ST, et al. Diurnal fluctuations in corneal topography 10 years after radial keratotomy in the prospective evaluation of radial keratotomy study. *J Cataract Refract Surg*. 1999;25(7):904-910.
4. Kwitko S, Gritz DC, Garbus JJ, Gauderman WJ, McDonnell PJ. Diurnal variation of corneal topography after radial keratotomy. *Arch Ophthalmol*. 1992;110(3):351-353.
5. Barraquer J. Jose Ignacio Barraquer 1916-1998—obituary. *Am J Ophthalmol*. 1998;126(1):167-168.
6. Trokel SL, Srinivasan R, Braren B. Excimer laser surgery of the cornea. *Am J Ophthalmol*. 1983;96(6):710-715.
7. McDonald MB, Liu JC, Byrd TJ, et al. Central photorefractive keratectomy for myopia. Partially sighted and normally sighted eyes. *Ophthalmology*. 1991;98(9):1327-1337.
8. Pallikaris IG, Papatzanaki ME, Stathi EZ, Frenschock O, Georgiadis A. Laser in situ keratomileusis. *Lasers Surg Med*. 1990;10(5):463-468.
9. Azar D, Camellin M, Yee R, eds. *LASEK, PRK, and Excimer Laser Stromal Surface Ablation: Refractive Surgery*. New York: Marcel Dekker; 2005.
10. Mathers WD, Fraunfelder FW, Rich LF. Risk of LASIK surgery vs contact lenses. *Arch Ophthalmol*. 2006;124(10):1510-1511.
11. Shortt AJ, Allan BD. Photorefractive keratectomy (PRK) versus laser-assisted in-situ keratomileusis (LASIK) for myopia. *Cochrane Database Syst Rev*. 2006;19(2):CD005135.

2

Corneal Flap Versus No-Flap Refractive Surgery

LASIK, Intra-LASIK, and Sub-Bowman's Keratomileusis Versus Photorefractive Keratectomy, LASEK, and Epi-LASIK

There is a lot of debate about the safety and efficacy of flap treatments, which include laser-assisted in situ keratomileusis (LASIK) and intra-LASIK versus surface ablation. There are studies to defend both sides of the argument and refractive surgeons who stand behind these studies.

Another factor to consider is how hard it is to manage complications (Figure 2-1). For example, a patient with epithelial ingrowth following LASIK may not have any loss of best-corrected visual acuity (BCVA) but may require débridement of the ingrowth in order to avoid loss of BCVA. This scenario will not be reflected in standard reports in the literature. Advocates of surface ablation appreciate the simplicity of the resulting ocular surface.

There are a number of studies that report overall safety and efficacy of surface ablation and flap-based refractive surgery are similar while some reports find that one technique may be superior to another for various reasons.[1-5] It can be difficult to compare flap versus surface ablation techniques due to differences in lasers, laser ablation profiles, microkeratomes, medications, and surgeons. In addition, it is difficult to compare studies that are more than a few years apart due to the impact of changing technology.

When determining which technique to recommend, there are several things to consider. Risks, recovery rates, and patient expectations are some factors that may influence patient choice and surgeon recommendations. An individualized approach to patient management is necessary to tailor recommendations to each specific case.

CORNEAL BIOMECHANICS

The relationship between alterations of the corneal surface and curvature changes was empirically understood prior to the popularization of radial keratotomy (RK). With the Munnerlyn formula, the quantification of corneal ablation depth as it related to refractive change was established and was adept at predicting standard ablation results. More complex mathematics, including the Zernike polynomials and Fourier transform, were applied to the study and measurement of higher-order aberrations (Figure 2-2).

These more complex formulas have allowed for the development of more complex wavefront corrections (Table 2-1). However, the response to laser ablation is not quite that simple due to the

Anderson Penno EE. *Surface Ablation:
Techniques for Optimum Results (pp 15–32).*
© 2013 SLACK Incorporated.

Figure 2-1. Epithelial ingrowth following LASIK is more common following enhancements or flap complications such as button-hole. Stable epithelial ingrowth can be monitored; however, expanding ingrowth requires flap lift and débridement. (Reprinted with permission from Gimbel HV, Penno EE. *LASIK Complications: Prevention and Management.* 3rd ed. Thorofare, NJ: SLACK Incorporated; 2004.)

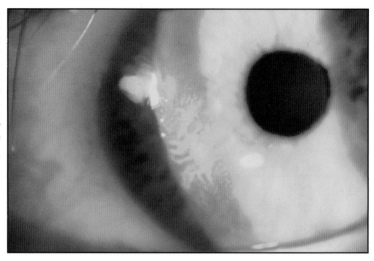

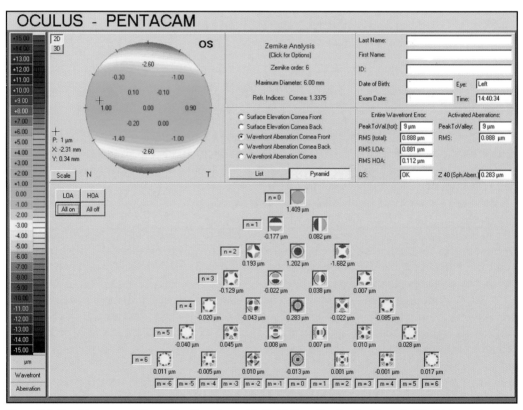

Figure 2-2. Graphic representation of Zernike polynomials that follows the standard format of the higher-order polynomials at the bottom with sequentially lower-order polynomials arranged in a vertical pattern.

TABLE 2-1. WAVEFRONT TERMS

Aberrometer	Device to measure higher-order optical aberrations of the eye.
Airy disc	The central bright region resulting from the diffraction pattern of a uniformly illuminated circular aperture.
Aliasing	A high-frequency pattern that is interpreted as a low-frequency pattern due to a frequency above the Nyquist limit of receptor sampling.
MTF	Modulation transfer function is the absolute value of optical transfer function.
Nyquist limit	The fundamental limit on special vision that results from the retinal mosaic density.
OTF	Optical transfer function is the Fourier transform of the object multiplied by the Fourier transform of the point spread function.
PSF	Point spread function is the distribution of light in the image plane for a point object.
PTF	Phase transfer function is the phase shift of image with respect to an object.
RMS	Root mean square is the standard deviation of the total wavefront with respect to ideal.
Strehl ratio	The theoretic amount of light contained within the Airy disc as a percentage of the theoretic maximum in a perfect optical system. Strehl ratio in a perfect system equals 1 and is less than 1 if wavefront errors are present.
Zernike polynomials	A series of mathematic formulas that are used to describe optical aberrations. They are often represented in a standard pyramid of graphics with each row representing the order of the polynomials from highest at the bottom to lowest at the top.

underlying biomechanics of the cornea and the effects of lamellar flaps or corneal thinning on corneal curvature. In addition, the cornea responds to the force in a nonlinear fashion due to the viscoelastic properties of the stroma.

The corneal stroma is approximately 80% water but this is not distributed equally throughout the cornea. The anterior stroma is less hydrated than the deeper stroma. The remaining percentages of stromal composition include 15% collagen and other proteins, salts, and proteoglycans. In addition, the peripheral cornea is thicker naturally and may become thicker in response to central ablation.[6] The anterior and peripheral stroma provides more mechanical strength than the posterior stroma, and the role of Bowman's membrane in corneal biomechanics has been debated.[7,8]

In addition to corneal hydration status, which can be a confounding factor in the study of corneal biomechanics and which is well known to impact surgical results, individual wound healing will also play a role in the final outcome of flap or no-flap treatments. The early hyperopic shift, which can be seen following surface ablation in particular, is in part due to the changes in the biomechanics of the cornea due to first central ablation and then surface remodeling over time.[9]

It is well established that both surface ablation and LASIK may result in a lowered measured intraocular pressure (IOP) postoperatively. Some studies have demonstrated a larger decrease in LASIK patients as compared to PRK 1 year after surgery.[10] This finding has been used to surmise that the corneas are weaker biomechanically following a lamellar flap than with surface ablation even when the final thickness is the same.

Creation of a LASIK flap without ablation will induce a hyperopic shift of a variable extent. This has likely been observed by most high-volume surgeons in cases where the flap was made but no ablation performed for a variety of reasons. This is another observed effect that indirectly demonstrates the biomechanical effect of flap creation. As a result of ectasia cases following LASIK, a push toward thinner flaps has resulted in the development of sub-Bowman's flaps.

The development of corneal hysteresis-measuring technology may provide a more direct measurement of corneal biomechanics both preoperatively and postoperatively. This technology may also aid in the screening of patients for keratoconus.

Although it may be tempting to assume that a lamellar corneal flap will always weaken the cornea to a greater extent than surface ablation, studies do not always support this theory.[11] For example, one study compared corneal hysteresis following LASIK to surface ablation with mitomycin C and found that the LASIK eyes had higher values; however, this study did not measure the preoperative corneal hysteresis values so the significance of this finding remains unclear.[12] The variability of results in studies that attempt to compare the biomechanical effects between different techniques reflects the complexities of the corneal response and the variety of techniques applied to laser vision correction.

Corneal cross-linking has been used increasingly in the treatment of keratoconus. Some surgeons recommend corneal cross-linking for suspicious topography. If the use of corneal cross-linking becomes a standard procedure similar to the use of mitomycin C, the biomechanical weakening and risk of ectasia may be reduced for all excimer laser ablation techniques.

ECTASIA RISK

Ectasia risk is one of the driving forces for the resurgence of surface ablation. Corneal thickness was identified as a risk factor for corneal ectasia within the first few years after the introduction of LASIK, and a minimum corneal bed thickness of 250 μm was adopted as a safe standard. It has become clear over the many years that corneal refractive surgery has been performed that corneal thickness is not necessarily the whole story when evaluating risk of ectasia.

During the past decade, there has been considerable debate about the minimum safe residual corneal bed and many surgeons prefer to leave 300 μm or more residual bed following LASIK or intra-LASIK. More recent studies confirm that residual bed thickness is just one factor to consider when assessing ectasia risk (Table 2-2).[13,14]

The development of technology to create thinner and more consistent flap thickness from case to case with sub-Bowman's keratomileusis and with the femtosecond laser allows for treatment of thinner corneas while maintaining the theoretically adequate residual bed thickness. As these thin flap techniques are relatively new, the risk of ectasia may become clearer over time. The hazard of thin flaps may be the increased risk for buttonhole and challenge of managing thin flaps in the case of flap shift.

Surface ablation has continued to be the treatment of choice for thinner corneas. It is interesting that there is no clear consensus as to the minimum residual thickness following surface ablation. Anecdotal reports indicate that preferred corneal thickness following surface ablation varies between surgeons and ranges from more than 400 to 350 μm or even thinner for some surgeons.

In addition to the discussion about residual bed thickness, there has also been debate over the safety of laser vision correction in thin corneas even when the minimum bed thickness can be respected. Many surgeons will hesitate to recommend any type of laser vision correction for corneas with pachymetry of less than 500 μm. There have been studies in the literature that suggest that surface ablation is safe in thin corneas and there is still considerable debate about preoperative corneal thickness and risk of ectasia.

TABLE 2-2. ECTASIA RISK

Preoperative pachymetry	Debate continues about the role of thin corneas in ectasia.
Residual bed thickness	No published guidelines in peer-reviewed literature for surface ablation.
Abnormal topography	Identified in peer-reviewed literature as a significant risk factor.
High myopia	Deeper ablation depth has been identified as a risk factor.
Younger age	According to the meta-analysis by Randleman et al,[19] it may be a risk.

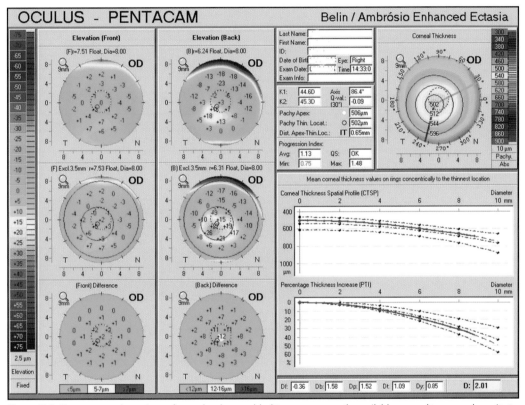

Figure 2-3. Keratoconus detection software has been added to many currently available corneal topography units to aid in the detection of forme fruste keratoconus.

A second recognized risk factor for ectasia following refractive laser ablation is abnormal topography. There have been advances in corneal mapping with the addition of keratoconus detection software for many units (Figure 2-3). For suspicious topography, many surgeons will advise surface ablation rather than LASIK. There are also increasing reports of PRK for the treatment of keratoconus.

In the past few years, PRK has been combined with corneal cross-linking and in some cases intrastromal corneal ring segments for the treatment of keratoconus. These developments are changing the recommendations for patients with abnormal topography.

TABLE 2-3. TOPOGRAPHIC KERATOCONUS DETECTION

INVESTIGATORS	METHOD
Rabinowitz YS, McDonnell PJ. *Refract Corneal Surg*. 1989;5:400-408.	Uses inferior superior (I-S) value to quantify I-S dioptric asymmetry.
Maeda N, Klyce SD, Smolek MK, Thompson HW. *Invest Ophthalmol Vis Sci*. 1994;35:2749-2757.	Used a number of indices to develop the Klyce/Maeda Index.
Smolek MK, Klyce SD. *Ophthalmol Vis Sci*. 1997;38:2290-2299.	Differentiates patterns of astigmatism, pellucid marginal degeneration, keratoconus, and contact lens warpage patterns.
Rabinowitz YS, Rasheed K. *J Cataract Refract Surg*. 1999;25:1327-1335.	Uses KISA% which is a product of K-value astigmatism index and skewed radial axis index.
Oshika T, Tanabe T, Tomidokoro A, Amano S. *Ophthalmology*. 2002;109:339-342.	Fourier analysis of topographic data.
Tanabe T, Tomidokoro A, Samejima T, et al. *Ophthalmology*. 2004;111:752-757.	Fourier analysis of topographic data.
Sato M, Kaji Y, Oshika T. *Ophthalmology*. 2004;111:752-757.	Enhanced ectasia detection tool using elevation.
Ambrosio R Jr, Belin MW. *J Refract Surg*. 2010;26(11):847-849.	Maps with best fit spheres and pachymetry data to identify corneas at risk.

Randleman and colleagues created a corneal ectasia risk score in their 2008 paper in the journal *Ophthalmology* by analyzing the literature available at that time.[15] The identified risk factors included abnormal preoperative technology, younger age, higher myopia, thinner preoperative pachymetry, and thinner residual bed thickness. Abnormal preoperative topography was the most significant risk factor according to this analysis, with residual bed thickness identified as the second most significant risk factor.

There have been many articles over the years that put forward indices to identify subclinical keratoconus (Table 2-3). These indices quantify inferior steepening and asymmetric bow-tie patterns along with pachymetry patterns to try to determine if these patterns fit forme fruste keratoconus. Keratoconus detection software in newer topography units can assist in the detection of abnormal corneas; however, other conditions such as anterior basement membrane dystrophy, significant dry eye, and corneal warpage may mimic subclinical keratoconus patterns.

Corneal hysteresis (CH) is gaining momentum as a screening tool to identify corneas at risk of ectasia, although, as with any new tool, more studies will need to be done in order to determine its use in preoperative screening. Measurement of CH involves using a rapid puff of air to create a corneal deflection. The inward and outward deflections are measured and a CH measurement is calculated. A low CH has been correlated with low-tension glaucoma and with forme fruste keratoconus. This technology shows promise as an additional tool to identify eyes at risk for ectasia following excimer laser ablation. CH may also be helpful in understanding the biomechanics of corneal flaps versus surface ablation.

At present, there is no single test that can reliably identify eyes at risk for ectasia (Figure 2-4). Ectasia following surface ablation is less common than post-LASIK ectasia, and there have been reports of ectasia developing following LASIK in one eye and not after surface ablation in the

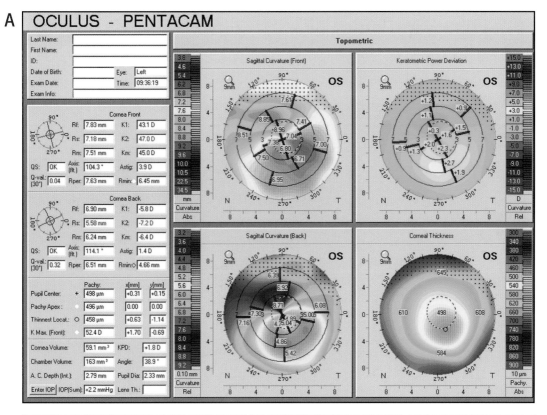

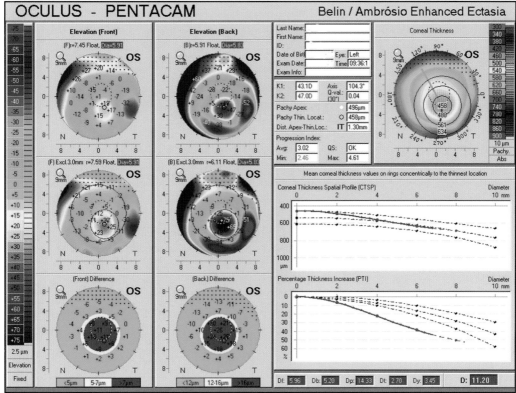

Figure 2-4. Ectasia is fortunately uncommon following corneal laser refractive ablation but can be very challenging to treat. Treatments include customized contact lenses, intrastromal corneal ring segments, corneal cross-linking, and corneal transplant.

TABLE 2-4. LASIK COMPLICATIONS	
Intraoperative	Flap complications (thin flap, partial flap, buttonhole), loose epithelium, decentered ablation
Early postoperative	Shifted flap, diffuse lamellar keratitis, infection, epithelial ingrowth
Late postoperative	Ectasia, late flap shift due to trauma

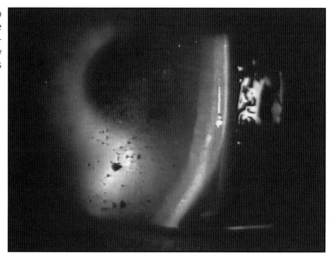

Figure 2-5. Although uncommon, flap complications can be challenging for the refractive surgeon to manage. Flap dislocation following LASIK can be particularly challenging if embedded foreign bodies are present.

fellow eye.[9] For this reason, surface ablation will continue to be a preferred choice in particular for eyes with higher-risk features, although ectasia has been reported rarely after PRK as well. Ectasia following surface ablation will also be discussed in Chapter 8.

FLAP COMPLICATIONS

Flap complications are an uncommon but well-known complication of LASIK and are another reason some surgeons and patients prefer surface ablation. There are a number of possible flap complications that can occur at the time of surgery, such as thin flap, partial flap, buttonhole, and loose epithelium (Table 2-4).

Other flap-related complications include shifted flap and diffuse lamellar keratitis. IntraLase (Abbott Medical Optics, Abbott Park, IL) has improved the predictability of flap thickness, but the overall safety and efficacy is equivalent to LASIK. While flap complications rarely result in loss of BCVA, they can delay healing or require additional surgery. Surface ablation techniques avoid the possibility of flap complications with the trade-off of longer recovery.

Dislocated flaps have been reported months to years after primary LASIK. Traumatic flap dislocation can occur from a variety of trauma from air bag injuries to more minor trauma, such as running into a branch while doing yard work (Figure 2-5). People with higher-risk occupations might prefer surface ablation to avoid the risk of traumatic flap complications. All patients should be counselled to wear safety glasses for any high-risk activities regardless of whether the patient has had refractive surgery.

Overall, the rates of flap complications between mechanical microkeratomes and femtosecond laser flap creation has been reported in some series to be similar, although reports are variable,

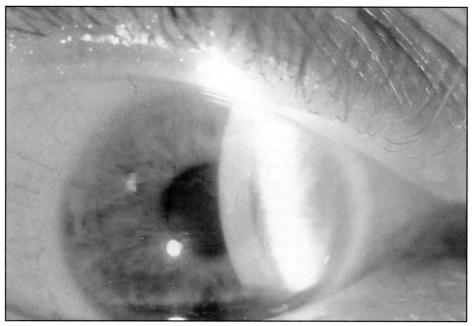

Figure 2-6. Loose epithelium over a LASIK flap. (Reprinted with permission from Gimbel HV, Penno EE. *LASIK Complications: Prevention and Management.* 3rd ed. Thorofare, NJ: SLACK Incorporated; 2004.)

indicating possible differences between surgeons or techniques. The advantage of the femtosecond laser is that, in many cases, a new flap can be made during the same surgical session.

As with any surgical technique, there will be a learning curve with newer technologies such that reported complication rates will be likely to decrease over time as experience is gained. Epithelial disruption may be more likely to occur following LASIK with a mechanical microkeratome (Figure 2-6); however, diffuse lamellar keratitis occurs with all methods of corneal flap creation.

Although best-corrected acuity can be maintained even with flap complications, it may require additional surgery. For flap procedures, there are several interfaces including the corneal surface, flap, flap interface with the stroma, and stroma. Managing complications such as buttonholes and loose epithelium over a flap can be challenging.

There is no flap with surface ablation, so the optical surface is simpler, which makes management simpler. Eliminating the flap avoids any possibility of flap complications or interface inflammation. There are increasing numbers of patients who specifically request surface ablation due to the possibility of flap complications with LASIK.

DRY EYE

Dry eye is the most common side effect of refractive surgery. Some studies suggest that LASIK is more likely to trigger more severe dry eye.[16] Attention to ocular surface disorders is imperative regardless of the refractive surgery technique considered. Many patients are motivated to have refractive surgery due to dry eye preoperatively. If surface disease is not identified and treated prior to surgery, then patients will likely blame their symptoms on the surgery.

Patients may be more sensitive to symptoms of ocular surface disease after refractive surgery simply because their eyes are more exposed. Spectacles provide protection against evaporation, airborne irritants, and wind. Contact lenses may diminish sensitivity due to the fact that the corneal surface is covered. Most patients, regardless of refractive surgery techniques, will experience more

TABLE 2-5. SURFACE ABLATION COMPLICATIONS

Intraoperative	Loose epithelium, decentered ablation
Early postoperative	Infection, slow re-epithelialization
Late postoperative	Ectasia, corneal haze

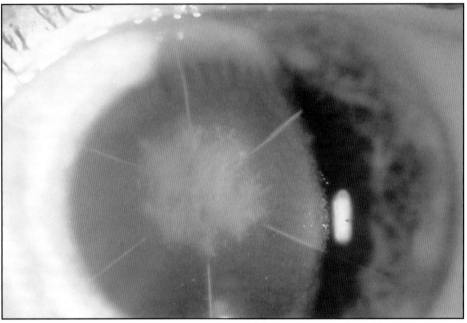

Figure 2-7. Visually significant corneal haze is uncommon following primary surface ablation but can occur even in cases where intraoperative mitomycin C has been used. Corneal haze is more likely to develop in high correction and when surface ablation is used following RK, LASIK, and other irregular corneal surfaces. (Reprinted with permission from Gimbel HV, Penno EE. *LASIK Complications: Prevention and Management.* 3rd ed. Thorofare, NJ: SLACK Incorporated; 2004.)

dry eye for some period of time after surgery or permanent increased sensitivity to environmental irritants, such as cutting onions, when their corrective lenses are discontinued.

There are new tools available to measure tear osmolarity that may be useful for preoperative screening. Schirmer's measurements can be highly variable and may not correlate with symptoms in some cases. Identifying, counseling, and treating dry eye patients before surgery appears to be a more important predictor of postoperative dry eye than whether a flap or no-flap technique is used for refractive correction.

CORNEAL HAZE

Risk of corneal haze was one of the driving factors in the rise of the popularity of LASIK in the 1990s (Table 2-5). Haze, in many cases, will be visible at the slit-lamp but will not produce visual symptoms. However, in severe cases, haze can lead to reduced best-corrected vision, halos, starbursts, and decreased quality of vision (Figure 2-7). Estimates of significant haze range from 0.5% to 5% with some series in the recent literature reporting no cases of visually significant haze.[12,17]

Improvements in laser technology have reduced the risk of visually significant haze, most notably with larger treatment zones compared to the early generations of excimer lasers. Variable spot size and variable repetition rate for broad-beam excimer platforms has been developed, which has been reported to improve accuracy of the ablation and reduce heat generation, which may contribute to haze. Scanning slit-lasers are anecdotally less likely to result in haze after surface ablation, and older studies indicated that the flying spot lasers are less likely to produce haze as compared to broad-beam lasers.[18]

There are suggestions that epithelial removal technique may influence haze development following surface ablation, but most studies conclude that these differences resolve over 3 to 12 months.[19] Corneal haze is a complication that is more likely to occur following surface ablation than LASIK. Sub-Bowman's keratomileusis and thin flap intra-LASIK would theoretically be less likely to produce haze but there have been sporadic reports of haze following these thin flap techniques, which some investigators believe may be due to disruption of Bowman's membrane.[17]

The use of mitomycin C for higher corrections has also reduced the incidence of visually significant haze. Some surgeons use mitomycin C at the time for treatment for all levels of corrections and others will use mitomycin C for higher corrections only. In particular, for hyperopic corrections and for higher myopic corrections, the use of mitomycin C should be considered for surface ablation. Haze can occur even with the use of mitomycin C, although it is uncommon.

For high myopic corrections and higher hyperopic corrections, LASIK has historically been recommended over PRK due to risk of haze. These recommendations may be changing as a result of the improvement in surface ablation techniques, including technological advances in ablation profiles and the use of mitomycin C, which has reduced the incidence of visually significant haze.

The risk of haze with newer thin flap techniques will become more apparent over time but at present, haze has not been widely reported as a result of these techniques. There have been isolated cases of haze following femtosecond LASIK. Vaddavalli and colleagues report a case with flap thickness of 73 μm and 81 μm.[20] On high-resolution optical coherence tomography (OCT), there were areas of Bowman's membrane disruption, which were correlated with the densest areas of haze.

WAVEFRONT

The ability to measure and record higher-order aberrations has led to the development of wavefront-optimized and wavefront-guided laser ablation platforms (Figure 2-8). These ablation patterns will be covered in more detail in Chapter 6. There has been debate about whether the corneal flap might mask the benefit of wavefront treatments.

The most commonly used aberrometers use infrared light to illuminate the fovea. The reflected rays are analyzed with a Hartmann-Shack array of micro lenses. The deviation of the reflected rays are measured and reported as a deviation from an ideal wavefront using a mathematical method called Zernike polynomials. The wavefront map can be used for wavefront-guided ablation for both flap and no-flap treatments.

Some surgeons believe that the results are best with a combination of wavefront and surface ablation techniques, although many studies do not show statistically significant differences between wavefront-guided ablations on the surface versus under a flap.

SURFACE ABLATION VERSUS FLAP FROM PATIENT PERSPECTIVE

Many patients have some information about refractive surgery options from talking to friends and family who may have had laser vision correction and from information they obtain on the

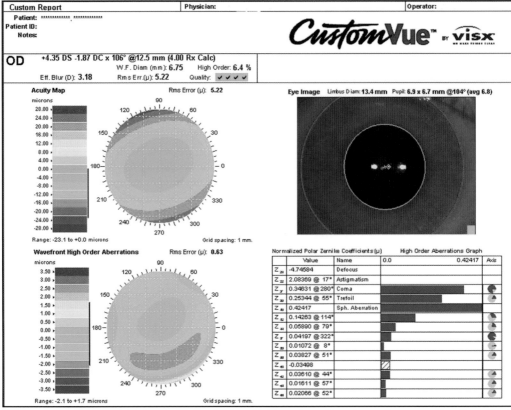

Figure 2-8. Wavefront aberrometers use infrared light, which is projected into the pupil space and is reflected back from the fovea. The reflected rays are measured by an array of lenses called a Hartmann-Shack array and are used to generate a wavefront map. (WaveScan system, Abbott Medical Optics Inc.)

TABLE 2-6. SURFACE ABLATION VERSUS FLAP FROM PATIENT PERSPECTIVE		
	SURFACE ABLATION	**FLAP**
Recovery	Longer with surface ablation	Shorter with flap treatment
Pain	Less discomfort during surgery More discomfort in first 23 days	More discomfort during surgery Less discomfort in first few days
Risk	Lower risk, haze possible	Higher risk of ectasia, flap complications
Enhancement	Possibility of enhancement	Possibility of enhancement
Outcome	Excellent	Excellent

Internet. Primary considerations are cost, recovery time, safety, and pain (Table 2-6). Only a few patients express specific concerns about the final outcomes of one technique over another.

Recovery is considerably slower in the first week with surface ablation compared to flap treatments, which can be an issue for patients who have limited time off of work, childcare duties, or

TABLE 2-7. SURFACE ABLATION VERSUS FLAP FROM SURGEON PERSPECTIVE

	SURFACE ABLATION	FLAP
Recovery	Longer with more chair time postoperatively	Shorter with flap treatment
Intraoperative	Simpler technique	More complex depending on method
Risk	Lower risk, haze possible Haze can be challenging to treat	Higher risk of ectasia, flap complications Complicated flaps can present challenges
Enhancement	Possibility of enhancement	Possibility of enhancement
Outcome	Excellent	Excellent

other daily responsibilities. Recovery time is also an issue for patients who may be trying to have surgery just before a big event, such as a wedding or a new job.

Even though flap-based laser ablation would be expected to provide excellent early results, it may be unwise to perform any type of refractive surgery just prior to a major event. Although uncommon, there is the possibility that there may be complicating factors such as dry eye or night vision disturbance in the early postoperative period even following LASIK or intra-LASIK.

Fear of pain can lead patients to avoid surface ablation or conversely to avoid a corneal flap due to the fear of intraoperative pain. In either case, explaining to the patient what to expect for both intraoperative sensations and during recovery will help to reduce anxiety. There is a lot of variability between patients in terms of intraoperative and postoperative experiences but, in general, anxiety will increase their perceptions of pain. Being realistic with expectations is particularly important with surface ablation during the re-epithelialization phase.

Many patients who request surface ablation specifically believe that it carries a lower risk. Some just do not like the thought of cutting a flap. Only a few patients are aware of ectasia and corneal haze. While patients are generally more informed due to access to the Internet, they will still need careful counseling and education about the potential risks and benefits presented in an understandable format.

SURFACE ABLATION VERSUS FLAPS FROM SURGEON PERSPECTIVE

For the surgeon and staff, surface ablation may require more chair time due to increased postoperative visits in the first week. There may be additional telephone calls with surface ablation patients in the first few postoperative days when discomfort is to be expected (Table 2-7).

Intraoperatively, surface ablation is simpler in general for the surgeon. Costs of surgery are likely to be lower with surface ablation depending on techniques. Femtosecond laser flap creation adds additional costs due to the need for a second laser and may take slightly longer if the patient is being moved between 2 lasers, first for flap creation then for excimer ablation.

While the risk of intraoperative complications is low, complications are more likely with LASIK or intra-LASIK due to flap creation. Flap complications can often be corrected but can involve more lengthy surgery time or repeat surgery, such as epithelial ingrowth removal.

During the first 3 to 6 months, surface ablation patients may need more reassurance as there are some patients who will have a slower recovery of quality of vision; however, some patients who have had a flap-based refractive technique complain about reduced quality of vision due to dry eye or night vision disturbance for weeks or months following surgery.

Postoperative flap complications, such as flap shifts, epithelial ingrowth, or diffuse lamellar keratitis, can be difficult to manage in some cases. Visually significant haze, although rare, can be challenging due to the fact that treatment is generally to use topical steroids for a number of months, and retreatment can only be considered when the vision and refraction are stable. Ectasia is fortunately uncommon with any corneal refractive surgery technique; however, it would be even more unlikely to develop after surface ablation.

Most surgeons will develop an array of techniques with which they are comfortable and that provide them with good outcomes. For some surgeons, the additional chair time required for

TECHNIQUES OF MECHANICAL EPITHELIAL REMOVAL

Ioannis Pallikaris, PhD, MD; Maria Kalyvianaki, PhD, MD; and Harilaos Ginis, PhD

Although photorefractive keratectomy (PRK) is considered to be effective and safe for the correction of refractive errors,[1] slow visual recovery and postoperative discomfort have made laser-assisted in situ keratomileusis (LASIK) the procedure of choice among refractive surgeons[2] and patients. However, risk of flap-related complications and corneal ectasia,[3] especially in thin corneas, have renewed surgeons' interest in surface ablations. The variants of advanced surface ablations are differentiated by the method of epithelial débridement before photorefractive corrections. In this chapter, the 2 main automated approaches (and representative devices) of mechanical epithelial removal prior to surface ablation procedures are presented.

Mechanical débridement of the epithelium with a blunt spatula—as originally employed in PRK—provides excellent surgical control. This method has been reported to create minor scratches on Bowman's layer.[4] Although these microscopic scratches are unlikely to have any clinical significance, this method requires longer surgical times and introduces variability to the procedure. These disadvantages led to the development of more automated techniques aiming to provide faster and more consistent epithelial removal.

All methods of mechanical removal of the epithelium are based on the different mechanical properties of the epithelium in comparison to the underlying collagen-rich tissue. In particular, the higher tensile strength of Bowman's layer (or corneal stroma) can provide a distinct cleavage plane without other means of limiting the penetration depth of any instrument that is designed to remove the epithelium.

THE ROTATING BRUSH

The first approach for automated epithelial removal was a rotating brush (Figure 2A-1). These devices are based on an early battery-operated device that was developed in 1993 by Pallikaris and coworkers.[8] This device featured a plastic disposable tip with flexible bristles made of polyethylene. The tip was rotated at about 2000 RPM by a DC electric motor. The device did not feature electronic control of the rotation speed as preliminary experiments demonstrated that this parameter was not critical for the effectiveness of the device.

These devices, including the commercially available "Amoils brush" (Innovative Excimer Solutions Inc, Toronto, Canada), rely on repetitive strokes from the fast-moving bristles to emulsify the epithelial layer without damage to the underlying Bowman's or stroma. This is achieved by using bristles of appropriate stiffness. Typically, epithelial removal is achieved over a diameter equal to that of the brush tip after 3 to 5 seconds of contact of the rotating tip with the cornea. Although there have been no measurements, it is hypothesized that no significant temperature rise is associated with the heat generated by the friction between the cornea and the brush.

These brushes have been evaluated microscopically and clinically[7,8] and have been shown to provide a smooth stromal bed and normal re-epithelialization times postoperatively.

Off-label use of electric dental brushes to remove corneal epithelium has been communicated in conferences; however, the safety of this practice has not been documented in an organized study.

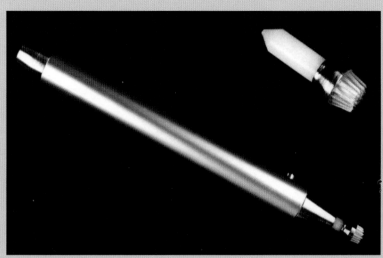

Figure 2A-1. Rotating brush.

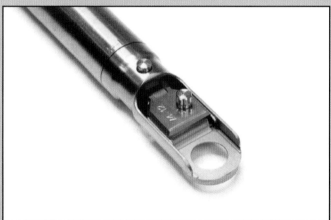

Figure 2A-2. Epikeratome.

EPIKERATOMES

In laser epithelial keratomileusis (LASEK), the epithelium is separated as a sheet with the use of alcohol solution on the cornea (Figure 2A-2). To avoid the use of alcohol, mechanical separation of the epithelial sheet with the use of a fully automated device, the epikeratome, was introduced as the epi-LASIK technique.[5] At the end of this procedure, the epithelial flap can either be repositioned on the ablated stroma or not (off-flap epi-LASIK[6,7]).

The epikeratome is a fully automated device that is designed to separate the epithelium from the stroma as a sheet. It comprises an oscillating specially designed blade, the forward movement of which separates the epithelial sheet. The principle of operation of these devices involves the use of a blade with appropriate edge design. These blades feature a facet (Figure 2A-3) sliding on the surface of the cornea. The direction of movement in combination with the shape of the blade's edge ensures that the blade does not penetrate the stroma. In contrary to the brushes, in these devices, the blade transverses only once across the cornea and the epithelium is separated as a complete sheet. In order to ensure proper contact of the blade's edge with the cornea and correct relative position of the blade and the free surface of the cornea, these devices feature a suction ring that increases the intraocular pressure to levels similar to that of LASIK microkeratomes. Removal of the epithelium with an epikeratome allows the surgeon to reposition the epithelium on the surface of the cornea after laser

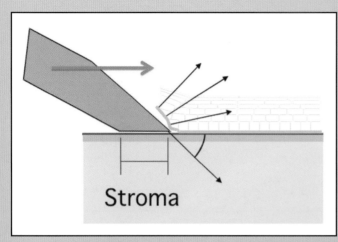

Figure 2A-3. Epikeratome blades feature a facet sliding on the surface of the cornea.

treatment. The effectiveness of this practice in terms of postoperative pain, rehabilitation time, and refractive outcome is disputed.[9,10]

The main disadvantage of the epikeratome device is its high initial and operational cost in comparison to the much simpler brush-based device.

The main advantages of epikeratomes as devices to remove the epithelium even if there is no surgical plan to reposition the epithelial flap after treatment is the consistent diameter of de-epithelialization and the very clean borders of the de-epithelialized zone. This characteristic has been anecdotally hypothesized to promote faster re-epithelialization.

Efficient and safe epithelial removal is not only a critical step in a successful surface ablation procedure, but is also an important parameter in patient flow and management of surgical time. The need for reproducible and efficient tools to remove the epithelium has led to the development of different mechanical devices. These devices in the future may be further improved in order to provide smoother borders of the de-epithelialized zone and even asymmetric (eg, elliptical) de-epithelialization zones in order to accommodate astigmatic ablations. The importance of these parameters cannot be elucidated before these steps are taken.

REFERENCES

1. Bricola G, Scotto R, Mete M, Cerruti S, Traverso CE. A 14-year follow-up of photorefractive keratectomy. *J Refract Surg.* 2009;25(6):545-552.
2. Sandoval HP, de Castro LE, Vroman DT, Solomon KD. Refractive surgery survey 2004. *J Cataract Refract Surg.* 2005;31(1):221-233.
3. Pallikaris IG, Kymionis GD, Astyrakakis NI. Corneal ectasia induced by laser in situ keratomileusis. *J Cataract Refract Surg.* 2001;27(11):1796-1802.
4. Griffith M, Jackson WB, Lafontaine MD, Mintsioulis G, Agapitos P, Hodge W. Evaluation of current techniques of corneal epithelial removal in hyperopic photorefractive keratectomy. *J Cataract Refract Surg.* 1998;24(8):1070-1078.
5. Pallikaris IG, Naoumidi II, Kalyvianaki MI, Katsanevaki VJ. Epi-LASIK: comparative histological evaluation of mechanical and alcohol-assisted epithelial separation. *J Cataract Refract Surg.* 2003;29(8):1496-1501.
6. Kalyvianaki MI, Kymionis GD, Kounis GA, Panagopoulou SI, Grentzelos MA, Pallikaris IG. Comparison of epi-LASIK and off-flap epi-LASIK for the treatment of low and moderate myopia. *Ophthalmology.* 2008;115(12):2174-2180.
7. Wang QM, Fu AC, Yu Y, et al. Clinical investigation of off-flap epi-LASIK for moderate to high myopia. *Invest Ophthalmol Vis Sci.* 2008;49:2390-2394.
8. Pallikaris IG, Karoutis AD, Lydataki SE, Siganos DS. Rotating brush for fast removal of corneal epithelium. *J Refract Corneal Surg.* 1994;10(4):439-442.

9. Kalyvianaki MI, Kymionis GD, Kounis GA, Panagopoulou SI, Grentzelos MA, Pallikaris IG. Comparison of epi-LASIK and off-flap epi-LASIK for the treatment of low and moderate myopia. *Ophthalmology.* 2008;115(12):2174-2180.

10. Wang QM, Fu AC, Yu Y, et al. Clinical investigation of off-flap epi-LASIK for moderate to high myopia. *Invest Ophthalmol Vis Sci.* 2008;49(6):2390-2394.

postoperative care is worth not having to manage the rare but potentially time-consuming, complicated flap patient.

SUMMARY

It can be confusing for patients to understand the pros and cons of different approaches. The explosion of acronyms used for both flap and no-flap treatments is adding to the confusion. For patients who qualify for both types of refractive surgery, the choice is ultimately up to them with their surgeon's guidance. The surgeon's role is to educate patients in order for them to make the choice that is best for their individual case. In some cases, the best choice may be to not have any refractive surgery.

LASIK and intra-LASIK continue to be the most commonly performed excimer laser refractive surgeries due to the rapid recovery of vision possible with these techniques, but there are an increasing number of people who are specifically asking for surface ablation in order to avoid the possibility of flap complications during or after surgery. With proper preoperative counseling and support during the early days following surgery, patients are willing to accept the inconvenience of slower vision recovery and more discomfort in the short-term to benefit from the excellent long-term results available with surface ablation.

There is a wider variety of techniques to choose from than ever before for both the refractive surgeon and patient. Weighing the risks and benefits of each technique is necessary for the surgeon to decide what range of techniques to offer. Many surgeons still offer flap options and reserve surface ablation for specific cases, such as thinner corneas. However, there are increasing numbers of refractive surgeons who only offer surface ablation due to the excellent results and low complication rates.

REFERENCES

1. Manche EE, Haw WW. Wavefront-guided laser in situ keratomileusis (Lasik) versus wavefront-guided photorefractive keratectomy (Prk): a prospective randomized eye-to-eye comparison (an American Ophthalmological Society thesis). *Trans Am Ophthalmol Soc.* 2011;109:201-220.

2. Hatch BB, Moshirfar M, Ollerton AJ, Sikder S, Mifflin MD. A prospective, contralateral comparison of photorefractive keratectomy (PRK) versus thin-flap LASIK: assessment of visual function. *Clin Ophthalmol.* 2011;5:451-457.

3. Pirouzian A, Thornton J, Ngo S. One-year outcomes of a bilateral randomized prospective clinical trial comparing laser subepithelial keratomileusis and photorefractive keratectomy. *J Refract Surg.* 2006;22(6):575-579.

4. Sia RK, Coe CD, Edwards JD, Ryan DS, Bower KS. Visual outcomes after epi-LASIK and PRK for low and moderate myopia. *J Refract Surg.* 2012;28(1):65-71.

5. Ghadhfan F, Al-Rajhi A, Wagoner MD. Laser in situ keratomileusis versus surface ablation: visual outcomes and complications. *J Cataract Refract Surg.* 2007;33(12):2041-2048.

6. Dupps WJ, Wilson SE. Biomechanics and wound healing in the cornea. *Exp Eye Res.* 2006;83(4):709-720.

7. Seiler T, Matallana M, Sendler S, Bende T. Does Bowman's layer determine the biomechanical properties of the cornea? *Refract Corneal Surg.* 1992;8(2):139-142.

8. Wilson SE, Hong JW. Bowman's layer structure and function: critical or dispensable to corneal function? A hypothesis. *Cornea.* 2000;19(4):417-420.

9. Lembach RG, Roberts C, Carones F. The refractive effect of the flap in laser in situ keratomileusis. *Invest Ophthalmol Visual Sci.* 2001;42(suppl 4):3235.

10. Hjordal JO, Moller-Pederson T, Irarsen A, Ehlers N. Corneal power, thickness, and stiffness: results of a prospective randomized controlled trial of PRK and LASIK for myopia. *J Cataract Refract Surg.* 2005;31(1):21-29.

11. Dawson DG, Grossniklaus HE, McCarey BE, Edelhauser HF. Biomechanical and wound healing characteristics of corneas after excimer laser keratorefractive surgery: is there a difference between advanced surface ablation and sub-Bowman's keratomileusis? *J Refract Surg.* 2008;24(1):S90-S96.

12. Wallau AD, Campos M. One-year outcomes of a bilateral randomised prospective clinical trial comparing PRK with mitomycin C and LASIK. *Br J Ophthalmol.* 2009;93(12):1634-1638.

13. Chan CC, Hodge C, Sutton G. External analysis of the Randleman Ectasia Risk Factor Score System: a review of 36 cases of post LASIK ectasia. *Clin Experiment Ophthalmol.* 2010;38(4):335-340.

14. Randleman JB, Russell B, Ward MA, Thompson KP, Stulting RD. Risk factors and prognosis for corneal ectasia after LASIK. *Ophthalmology.* 2003;110(2):267-275.

15. Randleman JB, Trattler WB, Stulting RD. Validation of the Ectasia Risk Score System for preoperative laser in situ keratomileusis screening. *Am J Ophthalmol.* 2008;145(5):813-818.

16. Hodge C, Lawless M, Sutton G. Keratectasia following LASIK in a patient with uncomplicated PRK in the fellow eye. *J Cataract Refract Surg.* 2011;37(3):603-607.

17. Sia RK, Ryan DS, Stutzman RD, et al. Alcohol versus brush PRK: visual outcomes and adverse effects. *Lasers Surg Med.* 2012;44(6):475-481.

18. Albietz JM, McLennan SG, Lenton LM. Ocular surface management of photorefractive keratectomy and laser in situ keratomileusis. *J Refract Surg.* 2003;19(6):636-644.

19. Pallikaris IG, Koufala KI, Siganos DS, et al. Photorefractive keratectomy with a small spot laser and tracker. *J Refract Surg.* 1999;15(2):137-144.

20. Vaddavalli PK, Hurmeric V, Wang J, Yoo SH. Corneal haze following disruption of epithelial basement membrane on ultra-high-resolution OCT following femtosecond LASIK. *J Refract Surg.* 2012;28(1):72-74.

Patient Selection and Preoperative Work-Up

Top 10 Red Flags

Preoperative work-up and preoperative patient counseling are the keys to excellent outcomes and satisfied patients. It is a challenge to maintain efficient use of clinic resources while ensuring a thorough approach. The investment of extra time in the patient selection and preoperative counseling process can avoid poor outcomes, unhappy patients, and more chair time postoperatively.

Following the telephone screening and in-office contact form, the topography and pachymetry are done at the start of the assessment at most centers as these are most often the disqualifying findings (Table 3-1).

Interestingly, spending time with a patient who is not a candidate to explain why can be your best tool to bring in prospective candidates. These noncandidates appreciate the time spent to identify risk factors and explain findings and will often refer additional patients to your practice as a result.

INTERNET AND TELEPHONE SCREENING

Internet

Most patients will use the Internet to research refractive surgery. In many cases, an Internet search will lead them to call a specific center and, in other cases, the patient may be referred to a center and use the Internet to find out more about the practice. A web site can be a useful patient education tool in addition to being used as a marketing device.

Having descriptions of the types of treatments offered along with pages on what to expect from various procedures can help the patient make a decision that is based on his or her individual needs and expectations. Information on who is a candidate and what factors may disqualify a patient from undergoing refractive laser ablation will reduce the number of noncandidates who call to book an assessment.

Referring the patient back to the web site can also be helpful following refractive assessment if the patient is looking for more information. There is a lot of information provided at refractive assessments and it can be hard for patients to remember it all. Many patients will appreciate even basic information on eye anatomy as they may not know how the eye works.

Anderson Penno EE. *Surface Ablation: Techniques for Optimum Results (pp 33-54).*
© 2013 SLACK Incorporated.

TABLE 3-1. PREOPERATIVE ASSESSMENT TESTING

Medical and ocular history	Intraocular pressure
Vision	Cyclorefraction
Manifest refraction	Slit-lamp examination
Corneal topography	Dilated fundus examination
Pachymetry	Special testing such as visual fields as indicated

TABLE 3-2. TOP 10 RED FLAGS

1. Systemic disease	6. Dry eye
2. Unstable refraction	7. Presbyopia
3. Thin cornea	8. Occupation
4. Abnormal topography	9. Inappropriate expectations
5. Eye disease	10. Specific contraindications

Patients should always be cautioned to consider the source of their information when using the Internet. Discussion boards and other types of web sites can contain incorrect information. It is important for the patient to also understand that refractive laser surgery is highly individualized, so even correct information may not apply to his or her case.

Telephone Screening

In most practices, potential refractive surgery candidates will either be referred or will call directly as a result of advertising. Having a thorough questionnaire for staff to use during phone calls can be a good screening tool and can avoid booking poor candidates for an assessment (Figure 3-1). There are several things that can often be identified during a phone call, which include systemic disease, changing refraction, refractions that are out of range, and inappropriate expectations (Table 3-2).

Many optometrists are well informed and will refer more suitable candidates. Providing seminars and educational materials to local optometrists can increase referrals of suitable refractive surgery candidates. It also is helpful for the optometrists to be familiar with the procedures offered and the range of corrections suitable. Even for the referred patient, the initial telephone call to schedule an assessment is an opportunity to gather key information and, in some cases, can identify a factor that will disqualify the patient from refractive surgery.

RED FLAG #1: SYSTEMIC DISEASE

Systemic disease has been discussed in the literature for decades as a potential risk factor for a poor outcome following refractive surgery (Table 3-3). In particular, collagen vascular disorders such as rheumatoid arthritis are considered to be a contraindication for any type of laser vision correction. History of iritis or other inflammatory eye disease may be risky.

New Patient Screening Form

Date _____ (d/m/yr) D.O.B. (d/m/yr) _____
_____Male _____Female   H.C. #_____

Patient Name _____

Address _____

City _____ Province _____ Postal Code _____

Home Phone _____ Work: _____ Cell: _____

Email:

Have you had a refractive assessment elsewhere? _____
How did you hear about W.L.E.A.? _____
Optometrist:_____

Circle Yes or No:
Do you have or have you ever had:

Rx if known	Yes	No	_____
Contact Lens Wearer?	Yes	No	Soft _____ Hard _____
Wear Readers?	Yes	No	_____
Diabetes?	Yes	No	Meds: _____
Rheumatoid Arthritis?	Yes	No	Meds: _____
Keloid Formations?	Yes	No	Meds: _____
Are you Pregnant?	Yes	No	_____
Are you Nursing?	Yes	No	_____
Autoimmune/deficiency?	Yes	No	_____
Allergies?	Yes	No	List: _____
Allergy to Latex/shellfish?	Yes	No	Airborne _____ Contact _____
Family Hx of Keratoconus?	Yes	No	_____
Are you taking Accutane?	Yes	No	_____
Are you taking Amiodarone?	Yes	No	_____
Hx of depression	Yes	No	_____

Occupation:_____

Hobbies: _____

Motivation for Refractive Surgery?_____

Office use:
- Quoted: $ per eye custom___
- Advised to leave contacts out   _____
- Advised to have a driver   _____
- Advised to bring sunglasses   _____
- Confirmation /PRK/Epi-LASIK Info sent_____
- Add patient to tracking sheet   _____

- ## Appointment scheduled for
- ## Initials _____

Figure 3-1. Telephone screening can be an effective tool for identifying factors that are contraindications for surgery. Using standardized checklists can be useful at all stages of the process.

TABLE 3-3. SYSTEMIC DISEASE AND SURFACE ABLATION

DISORDER	POSSIBLE RISK*
Collagen vascular disease	Possible corneal melt
Thyroid dysfunction	Risk of dry eye
Keloid scar	Haze
Diabetes	Refractive instability; slow re-epithelialization
	Possibly increased risk of infection
Systemic corticosteroid	Increased risk of cataract; risk of unstable refraction

*Each case must be considered on an individual basis. These are the most common systemic diseases, but this is not an exhaustive list and some of these associations have been debated in the literature.

Diabetes is not necessarily a contraindication for laser vision correction if the refraction is stable. There has been some discussion in the past regarding keloid scarring as a risk for corneal haze following photorefractive keratectomy (PRK) but it is not a strong association.

Pregnancy can affect outcomes both in terms of refractive stability and risk of haze following surface ablation. Ectasia triggered by pregnancy following laser-assisted in situ keratomileusis (LASIK) has been reported.[1] For these reasons, pregnancy should be included on screening questionnaires and, if a patient is actively planning to get pregnant, then consideration for deferring refractive surgery should be discussed.

Following pregnancy, nursing mothers should not undergo corneal refractive surgery until nursing is discontinued and normal menses resumes due to the possible effects on refractive stability and healing and also to avoid exposure of the infant to medications that may be prescribed to the mother.

RED FLAG #2: UNSTABLE REFRACTION

Unstable refraction can often be identified before the patient is booked for an appointment. When patients book an assessment, it is helpful to ask them to bring an old pair of glasses and to provide prior eyeglass prescriptions if available. Unstable refraction may be due to natural progression of myopia or astigmatism in patients in their teens or twenties. A stable refraction for at least 1 year and preferably 2 years is recommended for young patients.

Unstable refraction may also be an indicator of keratoconus if astigmatism is increasing (Figure 3-2). It can be helpful to do serial exams over a year or more to document refractive stability in younger patients or in patients with thinner corneas, topographic variations, or increasing cylinder.

If there has been a large myopic shift, consider checking a fasting blood sugar (Table 3-4). In patients who are 40 or older, an unstable refraction could indicate latent hyperopia or myopic shift due to early cataract. The cycloplegic refraction is a cornerstone of determining refractive stability. In particular, young high myopes may have progressive over-minus of their refraction, which may appear to be progression but on cyclorefraction is actually overcorrection. In some cases, young patients may have 1 D or even 2 D of overcorrection and not be affected by asthenopia. Latent hyperopia can also be identified on cyclorefraction. Latent hyperopes should be weaned into their full correction prior to laser vision correction. The presbyopic latent hyperope can be particularly difficult due to the fact that he or she will need readers regardless of correcting the hyperopia and may only be wearing glasses part time. Regardless of age, unstable refraction is a contraindication to refraction surgery.

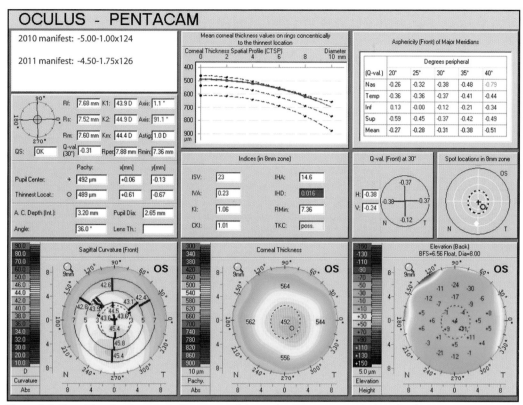

Figure 3-2. Unstable refraction may indicate corneal dystrophy. This patient was advised to have retesting in a year and subsequently was disqualified from corneal refractive surgery due to suspicious topography and increasing astigmatism.

TABLE 3-4. CAUSES FOR UNSTABLE REFRACTION

• Progression	• Corneal dystrophy
• Over-correction of myopia	• Corneal ectasia
• Latent hyperopia	• Cataract
• Diabetes	• Contact lens-induced corneal warpage

RED FLAG #3: THIN CORNEA

Surface ablation has been the mainstay for refractive laser correction in thin corneas for many years. Typically, patients with corneas that cannot support a LASIK flap and ablation with a residual bed of 250 μm or more have been recommended to have PRK. As some surgeons are moving to a thicker standard for residual bed thickness with LASIK, surface ablation is recommended more often for thinner corneas.

Some surgeons would not perform any laser ablation in corneas thinner than 500 μm; however, this standard continues to be under debate.[2] As discussed in Chapter 2, there are studies that demonstrate the safety of surface ablation in thin corneas. As there is not a consensus for residual pachymetry following surface ablation, careful consideration and thorough preoperative discussion with the potential candidate should be undertaken for patients with thin corneas who wish to undergo surface ablation.

RED FLAG #4: ABNORMAL TOPOGRAPHY

Abnormal topography is easy to identify when it clearly indicates keratoconus or pellucid degeneration, but there are a large number of patients who fall into a suspicious category with standard topography. In addition, ocular surface disease can lead to abnormal topographic patterns or variable topography. In more recent years, keratoconus detection software has been developed that can help identify early keratoconus (Figure 3-3).

Historically, keratoconus has been a contraindication to corneal refractive surgery. In an effort to reduce the risk of ectasia, patients with topographic abnormalities that are not severe enough to diagnose keratoconus but that may be forme fruste cases have been recommended to have surface ablation rather than LASIK. With the more recent addition of corneal cross-linking, some surgeons are treating keratoconus with combined cross-linking and PRK with good results.[3]

Contact lens over-wear can lead to topographic changes that may resolve with longer time out of contacts. Some centers only require 48 hours out of soft contact lenses and others will recommend a full week out of soft contact lenses prior to assessment. Rigid gas-permeable lens wearers may have to be out of lenses for 3 weeks or longer. For patients with suspicious topography and ocular surface disease or recent contact lens use, it is reasonable to ask them to stay out of their lenses longer and treat dry eye and blepharitis prior to repeating maps.

For patients with persistent mild topographic abnormalities, many surgeons will recommend surface ablation as a safer option to LASIK or intra-LASIK. It is important to discuss topography findings with the potential candidate due to the risk of ectasia. Ectasia is significantly less common after surface ablation but it has been reported in the literature.

RED FLAG #5: EYE DISEASE

Preoperative assessment will include a slit-lamp and dilated fundus exam. Many patients may not have had a complete eye examination in years or possibly may not have ever been dilated. A variety of conditions can be detected at the assessment, most commonly early cataracts, glaucoma, ocular surface disease, and corneal dystrophy (Table 3-5). While these conditions may not always be a contraindication to surgery, it is important to do a complete work-up with additional testing, such as visual fields, if needed, prior to surgery and to explain findings to the patient. There may be conditions such as severe surface disease or more advanced cataract that may be contraindications to laser vision correction.

Documenting existing eye disease prior to treatment will also eliminate the possibility that the patient will think that the surgery caused the eye disease. For example, if the patient has suspicious findings on optic nerve optical coherence tomography (OCT) with a normal field, explaining these findings preoperatively will be useful both to arrange appropriate ongoing surveillance and to make the patient aware that he or she is at risk for glaucoma in the future prior to having had laser vision correction. In some cases, pre-existing conditions, such as minor macular pigment changes, may not be contraindications for surgery but may affect the expected quality of vision.

Some patients present for refractive surgery and are found to have other ocular disorders. Glaucoma, cataracts, and dry eye are the most common disorders but more uncommon disorders such as retinitis pigmentosa are sometimes identified (Figure 3-4).

Special Testing

Special testing such as OCT and visual fields can be helpful in documentation and diagnosis (Figure 3-5). In many cases, there may be no treatment needed; however, a patient should be educated regarding any findings. Images from OCT testing can also be a useful tool for patient education.

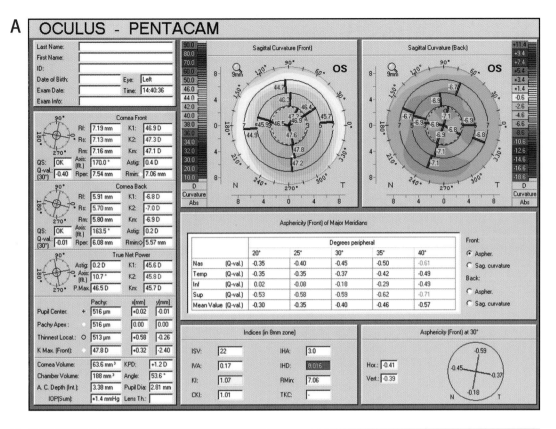

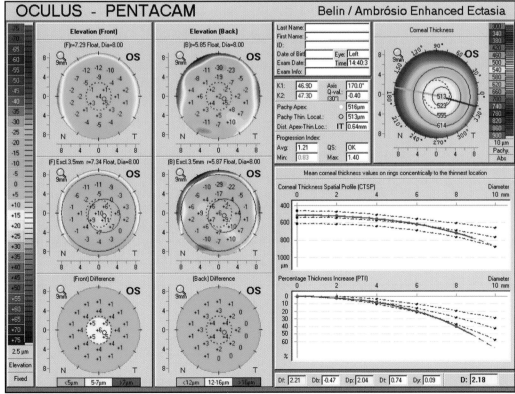

Figure 3-3. Keratoconus detection software will help in identification of abnormal topography.

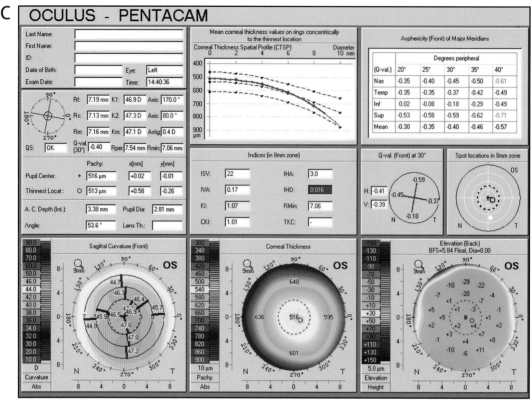

Figure 3-3 (continued). Keratoconus detection software will help in identification of abnormal topography.

TABLE 3-5. OCULAR DISEASE	
Dry eye	Dry eye may be worse in the first 3 to 6 months and the patient may be more symptomatic without lenses due to increased corneal exposure.
Glaucoma	May be identified for the first time at assessment. Topical medication may impact ocular surface.
Iritis	May pose a risk for recurrent inflammation or corneal melt.
Corneal scar	Risk of irregular astigmatism with epi-LASIK.
Herpes simplex virus	Herpes simplex keratitis may be reactivated.
Cataract	Can cause unstable refraction, reduced best corrected visual acuity.
Retinal disease	May result in reduced best corrected visual acuity.

A

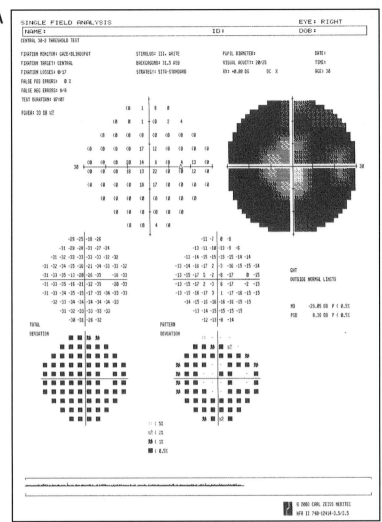

Figure 3-4. Retinitis pigmentosa (RP) diagnosed on refractive assessment, which included additional testing, is demonstrated in this figure. Following further consultations and education, the patient had PRK. Appropriate expectations, including an understanding of underlying RP symptoms and referral to community resources for assistance with visual disability, led to patient satisfaction with results.

RED FLAG #6: DRY EYE

Dry eye is a common presenting symptom in refractive surgery candidates. In some cases, the stated reason for wanting refractive surgery is contact lens intolerance. Most of these patients will have a combination of tear film deficiency and meibomian gland dysfunction, and some also have allergies. Treatment of these disorders usually involves time out of contacts, daily warm compresses, and daily artificial tears. Some patients may also need punctal plugs or topical cyclosporine for adequate correction of tear film abnormalities.

Tear film variations can also affect corneal topography (Figure 3-6). In some cases, the corneal topography may normalize after aggressive treatment of dry eye. Often, dry eye and possible contact lens warpage may be present on the initial examination. If repeat mapping is arranged, enough time should elapse between examinations in order to give the ocular surface time to improve.

Many people do not understand ocular surface disease and think that it will solve their problems if they can get rid of contact lenses with surgery. It can take a number of weeks or months in some patients to improve the ocular surface but it is well worth the chair time in order to avoid an unhappy postoperative patient who does not understand why his or her eyes are still uncomfortable and dry after laser vision correction.

Figure 3-4 (continued). Retinitis pigmentosa (RP) diagnosed on refractive assessment, which included additional testing, is demonstrated in this figure. Following further consultations and education, the patient had PRK. Appropriate expectations, including an understanding of underlying RP symptoms and referral to community resources for assistance with visual disability, led to patient satisfaction with results.

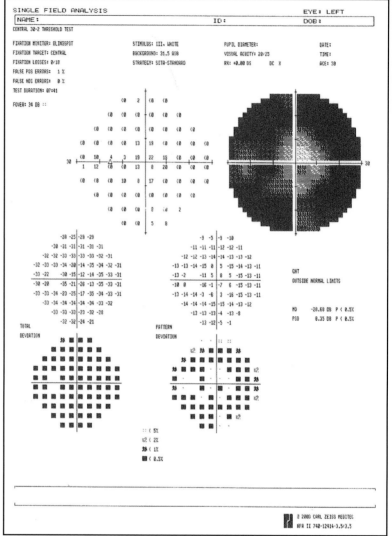

Some surgeons believe that the potential for severe dry eye or worsening dry eye may be more likely to occur after LASIK due to deeper disruption of the corneal nerves. There has also been some discussion of aberrant corneal nerve regeneration following LASIK, which can lead to chronic discomfort. Surface ablation may be less likely to trigger the worsening of dry eye due to the fact that corneal tissue is not affected as deeply. Most studies indicate that corneal sensation will recover to preoperative levels within the first few months for both LASIK and surface ablation patients.[4]

For dry eye patients undergoing surface ablation, careful preoperative counseling can help in preparing them for the postoperative recovery. Patients who have been wearing eyeglasses prior to surgery should be aware that their eyes will feel permanently drier due to the loss of the protection their glasses provide in reduced evaporation of the tear film. In addition to topical lubrication and warm compresses, frequent breaks from the computer or reading, oral flax and fish oil supplements, and eye protection with sunglasses when appropriate may be helpful.

Tear film dysfunction is a common condition in the immediate and intermediate postoperative period. For patients who are not managing well with topical lubricants, temporary punctal plugs

A

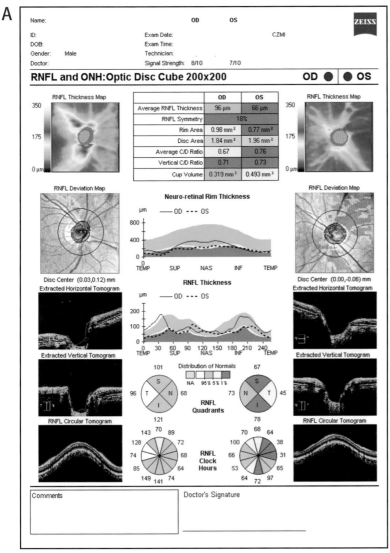

Figure 3-5. Glaucoma may be diagnosed in patients presenting for refractive assessment.

are a good option. These can be replaced if needed in the short term and if they are beneficial, then consideration for permanent plugs or punctal cautery can be discussed.

All dry eye patients should understand the need for consistent ongoing treatment in order to manage their condition. To avoid the unhappy postoperative patient, it is imperative he or she understands that laser ablation will not correct discomfort due to dry eye.

RED FLAG #7: PRESBYOPIA

Presbyopia can be another pitfall for refractive surgeons. In particular, the presbyopic patient who does not wear contact lenses may not understand the effects of full correction with laser ablation on his or her close vision. Contact lens wearers who are near presbyopic may struggle in particular in the first weeks or months following surface ablation as it can be common to measure up to a diopter hyperopic initially. For presbyopic patients who are wearing progressive lenses, it can be helpful to show full correction in a trial frame and give them small print to look at.

Figure 3-5 (continued). Glaucoma may be diagnosed in patients presenting for refractive assessment.

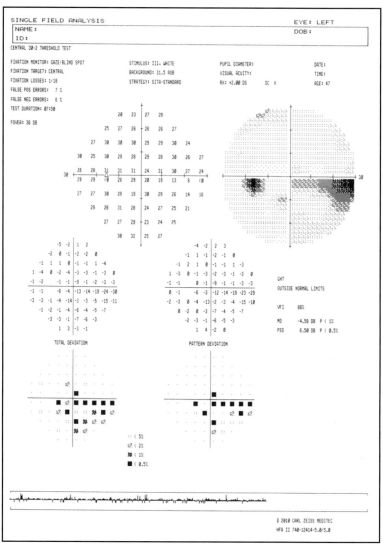

A discussion of activities that may involve a need for reading glasses can also be helpful. For example, patients may be unhappy if they need readers for activities like sewing or other close hobbies, putting on make-up, or doing fine crafts like woodworking. Patients in their fifth decade and older may need glasses for computer work. Many people have not thought about needing glasses for close work other than reading and may be disappointed postoperatively as a result.

Monovision can be a good compromise for presbyopes, but it is best if it can be tried in contact lenses prior to surgery. A trial frame demonstration can be done for noncontact lens wearers but it is limited in terms of real-life situations, such as night driving and prolonged computer work. As a rule of thumb, many providers recommend the dominant eye be corrected for distance; however, it is more beneficial to try it both ways as some patients will prefer the nondominant eye for distance. It is also important to counsel the patient that he or she may still need glasses for night driving or for very fine close work. Some surgeons will charge a fee to enhance an intentional monovision reading eye for distance correction. In this situation, it can be helpful to demonstrate to the patient with a trial lens or preferably with a contact lens trial the impact of treatment on close vision.

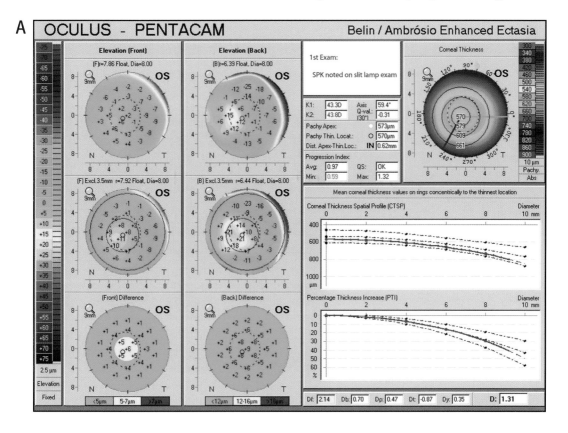

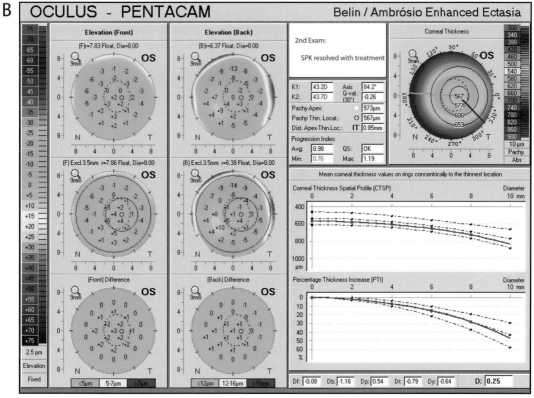

Figure 3-6. Dry eye can affect results of corneal mapping.

TABLE 3-6. VISUALLY DEMANDING OCCUPATIONS

- Pilot
- Law enforcement
- Paramedic
- Professional drivers
- Firefighters
- Surgeons
- Photographer

For presbyopes with mild myopia, a recommendation for no surgery or possibly to treat just one eye may be the best option. Presbyopic patients who present with mild myopia and a history of not wearing correction may be better off to continue as they are rather than sacrifice their close vision for distance correction with laser ablation. Once this is explained, many people will opt to not undergo laser vision correction.

RED FLAG #8: OCCUPATION

Occupations should be recorded as there may be specific requirements, such as pilots or firefighters for time off of work or for special testing such as color vision (Table 3-6). Many surgeons do not routinely test color vision as part of a preoperative assessment and for a patient undergoing laser vision correction for the purposes of a specific occupation such as firefighting, it will be a disappointment to find out after the surgery that he or she will not qualify. Some professions require postoperative contrast sensitivity testing before being cleared to return to work.

For pilots, ambulance drivers, professional transport drivers, and other visually demanding occupations, the safety of surface ablation may be appealing but the time away from work could be a factor to consider. The range for recovery of vision to the legal-to-drive range for a standard license ranges from a few days to 2 weeks, with most patients achieving uncorrected vision in the legal-to-drive range within the first week.

For occupations like driving and flying, the standards are more demanding and night vision disturbances can persist beyond the first few weeks. Although rare, complications from refractive surgery could cause a patient to no longer meet their occupational vision standards.[5]

Patients who have chosen surface ablation or are recommended to have surface ablation due to thin corneas or topographical changes need to be carefully counseled as to the potential range of time off of work that may be needed. In some cases, additional postoperative documentation may be needed for the patient to return to work or if the patient needs more time for vision recovery than expected. Supporting the postoperative surface ablation patient with this type of documentation will improve his or her satisfaction.

Many occupations require long hours on the computer. Dry eye, hyperopia in the early stages of healing, and visual aberrations that can be induced by a persistent fusion line will often lead to particular complaints relating to computer work. Many people want to return to work as soon as possible, and some will try to do work at home on the computer during the first few days following surface ablation in spite of recommendations to avoid it.

TABLE 3-7. INAPPROPRIATE EXPECTATIONS

- Eliminate reading glasses
- Improve best-corrected vision in amblyopia
- Correct dry eye
- Improve night vision
- Expect to return to work within 1 to 2 days following surface ablation
- Avoid any risks associated with refractive surgery

RED FLAG #9: INAPPROPRIATE EXPECTATIONS

Inappropriate expectations can be easy to identify in some cases and very hard in others (Table 3-7). In the initial telephone call, expectations such as a presbyope who wishes to eliminate readers or an amblyopic patient who wishes to improve best-corrected vision can often be discussed without bringing the patient in for assessment. Other common issues are contact lens-intolerant patients who do not understand the underlying ocular surface disease and patients who are looking for sharper vision than they are able to achieve with glasses or contact lenses.

For surface ablation, a very common inappropriate expectation is related to the time required for vision recovery. Most people can understand the first few days when the bandage contact lens is in place, but often they will underestimate the time needed off of work. In spite of careful preoperative counseling, some patients will be frustrated in the first few weeks or months with the quality of vision, with fluctuating vision, or with night vision effects. Some people wish to schedule refractive surgery just before getting married, starting school, traveling, or before beginning a big project at work. If possible, potential surface ablation candidates should be counseled to give themselves enough time for recovery before these types of activities.

In some cases, in spite of thorough preoperative discussions, the patient has surface ablation surgery just before starting a new job, university, or some other demanding activity. These situations can be stressful for the surgeon and the patient and will require more postoperative visits and possibly more paperwork in order to help the patient during the recovery of vision. It is not always possible to identify the patients who will have difficulty dealing with the fluctuations of vision that may be present for weeks or months following surface ablation.

Red flags include people who complain they frequently have to change their glasses and have a hard time getting their lenses made correctly (Table 3-8). Patients who have difficulty scheduling preoperation or surgery, or patients who say they cannot afford to take time off of work for postoperative appointments due to frequent scheduling conflicts could present challenges. Extreme anxiety about possible complications may indicate that the patient will have difficulty tolerating the longer visual recovery of surface ablation.

Another potential problem patient is the person who asks no questions, is falling asleep, or is texting during the preoperative assessment. These patients may not be listening to the information provided and are likely to underestimate the healing process following surface ablation. In some cases, patients present for surgery and have not read the consent. It is imperative for patients to read the consent, and these patients may not be taking the risks of surgery and the recovery needed seriously.

If at all possible, identifying inappropriate expectations before surgery can avoid a lengthy postoperative course trying to manage the failed expectations in spite of a normal postoperative course. Unfortunately, it is not possible to identify every person with inappropriate expectations

TABLE 3-8. RED FLAGS FOR INAPPROPRIATE EXPECTATIONS

- Booking surface ablation just prior to a major event, such as wedding, new job, or travel
- Patients who say they do not have enough time for recovery or postoperative exams
- Difficulty in scheduling appointments
- Extreme anxiety regarding potential complications
- Failure to read informed consent and other educational material
- Texting or falling asleep during preoperative counseling
- Complaints of needing frequent prescription updates
- Chronic dissatisfaction with corrective eyewear

and in those cases, frequent postoperative visits to provide support through the first weeks to months is necessary.

Quality of Vision

If patients understand before undergoing surgery that it can take several weeks or, in some cases, several months to achieve their best quality of vision, then they will be less anxious or unhappy during the first few months. It can help to set a specific period of time after which enhancement might be considered. For example, some surgeons will not consider enhancement for at least 6 months and may recommend a longer interval for high corrections.

Surface ablation patients will often complain of ghosting, fluctuations of vision, monocular diplopia, and blurred vision within the first days to weeks following surgery. Some patients may need additional chair time to explain the healing process and expectations for recovery in spite of having spent time explaining these factors before surgery. There are a few people who will need additional time off of work or modified work duties following surface ablation.

Patients who live in rural areas or travel to and from work at night may need to find alternate transportation for some period of time as night vision may take longer to improve. This should be discussed before surgery, if possible. Attention to the specific vision needs for each individual can help guide the preoperative discussion and prepare the patient for the recovery following surface ablation.

Reassurance in the days and weeks following surface ablation is also important as a minority of patients will complain about quality of vision for weeks to months following surface ablation. Many of these concerns will resolve over weeks to months and, in some cases, an enhancement may be recommended after the refraction has stabilized.

RED FLAG #10: SPECIFIC CONTRAINDICATIONS

Specific contraindications to surface ablation include definite abnormal topography, unstable refraction, certain systemic diseases such as rheumatoid arthritis or other inflammatory diseases, past history of iritis, and unstable eye disease, such as changing cataract. Diabetics, glaucoma patients, and patients with significant ocular surface disease should be carefully screened for suitability. For epithelial laser in situ keratomileusis (epi-LASIK), contraindications include corneal scarring and prior corneal refractive surgery.

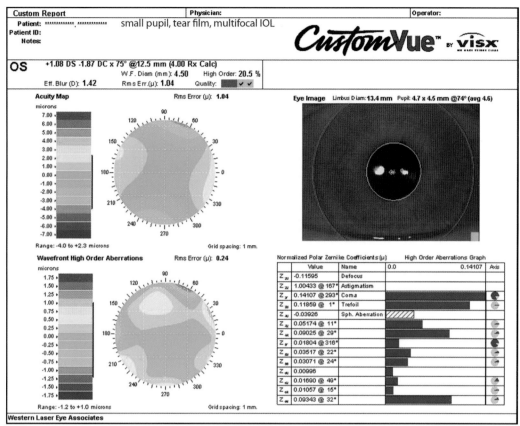

Figure 3-7. Small pupils may not be recommended for wavefront-guided ablation. (WaveScan system, Abbott Medical Optics Inc.)

Pupil Size

Pupil size should be discussed with patients if they have large scotopic pupils. Although the relationship between pupil size and night vision disturbances postoperatively has been under debate for decades, a patient with large pupils should be advised of this finding. Pupil size may also be an issue for wavefront-guided ablation (Figure 3-7).

Larger pupils can interfere with the ability for iris recognition in platforms that use this technology. Pupils smaller than 5 mm may also pose issues as there will be a smaller area of aberrometry data collected due to the small pupil area.

Psychiatric Conditions

Psychiatric diagnosis is not necessarily a contraindication to refractive surgery if the patient is stable and treated appropriately if treatment is necessary.[6] There have been reports that patients with depressive symptoms are more likely to be dissatisfied with refractive surgery and that this persists past 6 months postoperatively.[7]

Adding a question about past or present depression to preoperative questionnaires may be helpful in screening patients. If there is an indication of depression or other psychiatric condition, it is reasonable and important to discuss with patients how they think they would manage if there was a complication. Although complication rates are low, if a patient has a loss of best-corrected vision or quality of vision, it is a factor he or she may have to live with going forward.

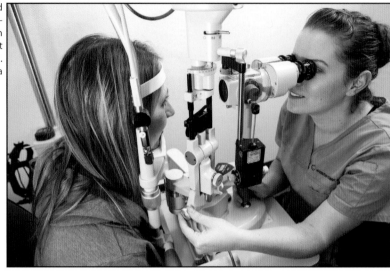

Figure 3-8. Educated staff are an asset to refractive practices and play an important role in patient education and counseling. (Photograph by Amanda Sneddon.)

There are no current guidelines for psychiatric screening of refractive surgery patients. Pre-existing depression or other psychiatric conditions may not necessarily be diagnosed but could make it more difficult for a patient to cope with possible complications or side effects of refractive surgery.

PATIENT EDUCATION

It can be helpful to review all the refractive surgery techniques available to the patient even if your practice may not offer all the options. By doing so, the patient is more aware of the variety of risks and benefits and can be more confident in his or her choice. For many patients, it can be helpful to have assessments at different centers in order to compare prices, options, staff, and surgeons. Patients who have taken the time to do more than one assessment are often more informed and more confident with their choices and are more likely to have the right expectations following surface ablation.

Some patients will need more reassurance and re-education in the early postoperative period that things will improve over time. Interim glasses may be helpful for some people if they are too early to consider enhancement, although this is rarely needed. Reminding patients that enhancement may be considered in the future can also reduce anxiety.

COMMUNICATION

Good communication skills are necessary for the staff and physician. Allowing enough time for discussion at the preoperative visit is critical. At most centers, the majority of the assessment will be spent with technical staff who will be performing the testing (Figure 3-8). An educated technical staff is a great asset to the physician for patient education.

It is helpful to provide patients with a pad of paper and pen at the start of the assessment in order for them to write questions down as they go along. Some patients will come to the assessment with a list of questions. There are some question lists online that include things like how many cases a surgeon has done and whether the doctor has ever been sued. In most cases, the technical staff may be able to answer the majority of the questions and defer to the physician to answer at the end of the assessment during the eye examination.

Sitting while talking to a patient has been shown to increase the perceived amount of time that is spent and provides the assurance that staff and physicians are taking the time to listen and answer all questions. Providing a quiet area for the potential refractive surgery patient to sit while viewing educational DVDs or reviewing other materials will help him or her to concentrate on the information being provided.

Booking an additional appointment time for discussion may be necessary for some patients who are undecided or may need to do a contact lens trial for monovision. Additional appointments are sometimes needed for a demonstration of monovision with a trial frame in noncontact lens wearers or to discuss the outcome of additional testing. If the patient is rushed and does not view the educational materials at the assessment, then a return visit should be scheduled so as to be sure he or she receives all the required information.

Clarification of a follow-up plan might be necessary if the patient will be comanaging with another optometrist or ophthalmologist for postoperative care. In particular, the timing of the first few visits and who will be removing the contact lens once re-epithelialization occurs should be discussed.

For new staff, it is helpful for them to sit in with more experienced staff to learn what information should be provided and to see how an experienced staff member handles various questions. Role playing between experienced and inexperienced staff can be a good tool to teach junior staff and build confidence in communicating effectively with patients.

OFFICE EFFICIENCY

As noted previously, office efficiency can start even prior to the first appointment. Effective use of telephone screening and an informative web site can reduce the number of calls for inappropriate candidates, such as the presbyope who wishes to get rid of reading glasses. Optometric outreach and education will also be effective in aiding the optometrist in forwarding candidates who are more likely to benefit from refractive surgery.

Refractive assessments can be time consuming for both the patient and the staff. It is imperative for the patient to be aware of how much time is necessary and to be prepared for a dilated examination with sunglasses and transportation from the appointment. Patients who present for refractive surgery are often highly busy and sometimes will arrive late or be rushed due to subsequent appointments.

An office policy, such as if the patient is more than 15 minutes late then only the undilated portion of the testing will be done and the patient will have to return for cycloplegic refraction and dilated examination, should be in place. This avoids any confusion on the staff's part and eliminates the domino effects a late patient can have on the remainder of the clinic schedule. Forewarn patients when booking an assessment that they should notify the office if they are going to be late for the appointment and that they may have to return for a second appointment if they are late.

Education and training of the staff will reduce the need to repeat testing. An educated staff will also be able to make the examining ophthalmologist aware of abnormal testing so the decision can be made if the assessment should be cut short if the patient is not a candidate (Figure 3-9).

A checklist can be helpful for both technicians and physicians to use during the preoperative examination and discussion (Figure 3-10). Just as aviators use checklists during the pre-flight checklist, refractive centers can benefit from their use in order to ensure that all information needed is recorded and that the discussion is complete. This form can also be used as a communication tool between technical staff and surgeon by noting any specifics regarding findings or expectations on the form, which can be passed along with the file when the technician testing is complete.

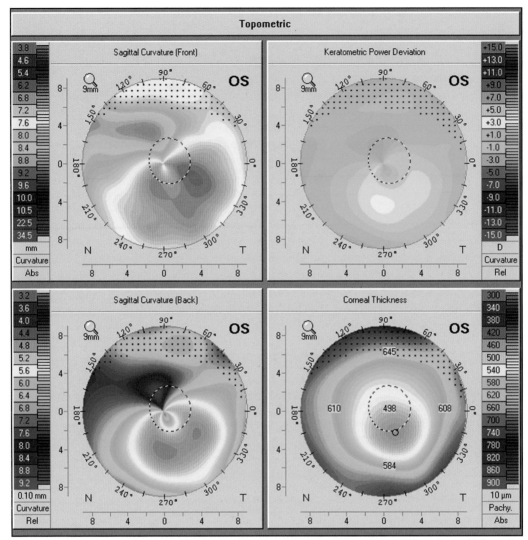

Figure 3-9. Pellucid pattern found on refractive assessment. Topographic abnormalities are the primary risk factor for the development of ectasia following refractive laser ablation. Significant abnormalities can be easy to detect while more subtle variations from normal may benefit from keratoconus detection software analysis.

For most patients, the postoperative course will be uncomplicated and postoperative visits will be straightforward and simple. Scheduled telephone calls in between visits can be useful and can reduce the in-office chair time and reduce extra appointments. In some cases, advice can be given as to pain management, dry eye treatments, and other matters without having the patient come to the office. This is a convenience to both the patient and office.

In complicated cases or unhappy postoperative patients, booking extra time with the surgeon or another examining ophthalmologist may be necessary. Booking these appointments at the end of the morning or afternoon allows for extra time without causing a back-log for subsequent clinic appointments.

Competent staff is the most important part of an efficient office. Patients appreciate being taken for their appointments on time and can recognize the expertise of educated technicians. Staff can also help keep the clinic flow on track by notifying the ophthalmologist of unexpected results at the assessment and on subsequent visits.

Refractive Counsellor Duties

New Patient Checklist:

__ Complete telephone referral form with the patient while on the phone

__ Enter information and start a chart

__ Book Ref Assessment appointment (4 consecutive ref assess time slots)

__ Mail a confirmation letter with surgery information sheets

- Appt Confirmation (print first page on letterhead)

- Make a copy of the confirmation letter for the chart, note in pt chart that patient information was sent.

__ OR Email to patient

- send email to patient with confirmation letter, surgery information; make sure to attach the PDF files only when emailing documents.

- transfer into patient file under referrals out.

__ Note on the tracking sheet how the patient found out about center

__ Check off on Referral Form if you have sent out patient information and that you have added Pte to tracking sheet and have quoted the surgery costs.

__ Scan copy of New Patient referral form into patients chart, put under intake & forms

__ Confirm Refractive Assessment appointments one day prior to the appointment date

Counselling:

__ Show the patient the DVD (always plug into power source after each Patient)

__ Ask if the patient has any unanswered questions.

__ Quote the surgery fees

__ Discuss scheduling of surgery

__ Show the pt the laser suite if they wish to see it.

__ Let the patient know they can call at any time for more information.

__ Give them a WLEA Brochure, CustomVue brochure, a Medicard pamphlet, FAQ and a business card to take with them.

__ Fill out "Refractive Pt Check List" and put in binder, check off where needed.

Figure 3-10. Checklists can assist in communication between staff and can ensure the work-up is thorough.

Summary

The initial screening begins with the first telephone call. Questionnaires can be used at the initial telephone call and at the preoperative screening to identify contraindications for surgery. Starting with topography and pachymetry will rule out some patients at the start of the assessment. Ideally, the surgeon should examine the potential patient at the preoperative assessment but if this is not possible, then the surgeon should communicate with the optometrist or ophthalmologist who is doing the preoperative assessment to be sure he or she is aware of the specific contraindications to surgery.

The preoperative assessment is a good time to communicate proper expectations and address any high-risk features. If possible, it can be helpful for the surgeon to address any high-risk features prior to the day of surgery to avoid having that conversation on the day of surgery or to avoid canceling on the day of surgery.

A thorough preoperative examination requires some investment of time on the part of patients and staff but it is well worth it. Good preoperative screening and counseling will lead to better outcomes and more satisfied patients.

References

1. Hafezi F, Koller T, Derhartunian V, Seiler T. Pregnancy may trigger late onset of kerectasia after LASIK. *J Refract Surg.* 2012;28(4):242-243.
2. Kymionis GD, Bouzoukis D, Diakonis V, et al. Long-term results of thin corneas after refractive laser surgery. *Am J Ophthalmol.* 2007;144(2):181-185.
3. Tuwairqi WS, Sinjab MM. Safety and efficacy of simultaneous corneal collagen cross-linking, with topography guided PRK in managing low-grade keratoconus; 1 year follow up. *J Refract Surg.* 2012;28(5):341-345.
4. Dooley I, D'Arcy F, O'Keefe M. Comparison of dry-eye disease severity after laser in situ keratomileusis and laser-assisted subepithelial keratectomy. *J Cataract Refract Surg.* 2012;38(6):1058-1064.
5. Davis RE, Ivan DJ, Rubin RM, Gooch JM, Tredici TJ, Reilly CD. Permanent grounding of a USAF pilot following photorefractive keratectomy. *Aviat Space Environ Med.* 2010;81(11):1041-1044.
6. Ortega-Usobiaga J, García-Sáenz MC, Artaloytia-Usobiaga JF, Llovet-Osuna F, Beltrán-Sanz J, Baviera-Sabater J. Myopic LASIK in psychiatric patients. *Cornea.* 2012;31(2):150-154.
7. Morse JS, Schallhorn SC, Hettinger K, Tanzer D. Role of depressive symptoms in patient satisfaction with visual quality after laser in situ keratomileusis. *J Cataract Refract Surg.* 2009;35(2):341-346.

Epithelial Removal Techniques
Photorefractive Keratectomy, LASEK, Epi-LASIK, Transepithelial Photorefractive Keratectomy

In the 1990s, the choices were much simpler: photorefractive keratectomy (PRK) or laser-assisted in situ keratomileusis (LASIK). With the advances in corneal refractive surgery over the past decades and the influences of marketing, the choices have exploded into an alphabet soup of techniques: PRK, LASIK, laser epithelial keratomileusis (LASEK), epithelial laser in situ keratomileusis (epi-LASIK), intra-LASIK, advanced surface ablation (ASA), keratome-assisted surface ablation (KASA), sub-Bowman's keratomileusis (SBK), and more (Table 4-1). Added to this are the additional intraocular options of multifocal intraocular lenses (IOLs), accommodative IOLs, phakic IOLs (implantable contact lenses, therapeutic contact lenses), and the list continues.

For the prospective laser vision correction patient, it can be helpful to categorize their options into simpler terms: flap or no flap. In general, the no-flap treatments involve a longer recovery but eliminate the risk associated with a corneal flap and the flap treatments allow for more rapid recovery of vision but may pose additional risks related to the corneal flap. Once patients understand that simple division into the 2 categories, they will understand that all surface ablation techniques involve removing the epithelium and the main differences in surface ablation techniques are how the epithelium is removed.

As the techniques of epithelial removal have evolved, there has also been some confusion as to what these techniques have been called in the literature. For example, alcohol-assisted epithelial removal has been used for decades for PRK, and yet in some reports this is called LASEK with flap removal. Over the past decades, there have been a few reports about using the excimer laser for epithelial removal.

While transepithelial laser ablation has not been commonly reported in the past several years, there has been renewed interest in this technique recently. More commonly, the routine methods of epithelial removal all use some variation of a mechanical method using dilute alcohol, corneal brush, or epikeratome.

PREOPERATIVE COUNSELING AND SLIT-LAMP EXAM

On the day of surgery, staff will spend some time with the patient reviewing what to expect during surgery and going over the postoperative instructions. At this time, preoperative drops are

Anderson Penno EE. *Surface Ablation: Techniques for Optimum Results (pp 55-66).* © 2013 SLACK Incorporated.

TABLE 4-1. CORNEAL REFRACTIVE SURGERY TECHNIQUES	
NO FLAP	**FLAP**
PRK/ T-PRK	LASIK
LASEK	Intra-LASIK
Epi-LASIK	SBK

given, which generally include a broad-spectrum antibiotic and a nonsteroidal anti-inflammatory. During this discussion, the staff will confirm that the patient has read the surgery consent, and if he or she has not read it, then time will be provided to be sure he or she has read and understood the information prior to signing.

It is a good habit to examine the patient at the slit-lamp in order to ensure that the cornea is clear prior to surgery. LASIK flap complications have been reported as a result of failure to recognize that patients had their contacts in at the time of surgery.[1] While it is uncommon to have a significant finding at this preoperative slit-lamp examination, it is an opportunity for the patient to ask the surgeon any final questions he or she may have.

At this time, the surgeon will also generally sign the consent form and add any additional notes to the standard consent forms if needed.

PHOTOREFRACTIVE KERATECTOMY

PRK is the original surface technique performed as early as the 1980s in the United States. Initially, the epithelium was removed using a beaver blade without the use of dilute alcohol. This method was more time consuming and could lead to either an irregular surface or to corneal desiccation. Original techniques recommended that the epithelium be removed from the peripheral treatment zone first in order to prevent central desiccation.

As techniques advanced, the 2 most common methods of epithelial removal for PRK involved the use of dilute alcohol and a well to contain the solution within a specific zone and the corneal brush. These 2 methods remain in use today.

Photorefractive Keratectomy With Dilute Alcohol

Dilute alcohol works by breaking the desmosome bonds between the epithelial cells and Bowman's membrane. There are variations of this technique but in general, a dilute solution (50% ethanol) is placed in a well of a specific diameter and is held in place to bathe the corneal epithelium in the treatment zone for approximately 10 to 20 seconds (Figure 4-1). Some surgeons use a blunt cannula to drip the alcohol solution into the well and others will soak a surgical spear in the dilute alcohol and then squeeze it onto the central epithelium. If surgical spear is used, it should be trimmed first in order to fit within the diameter of the well to avoid alcohol outside the intended treatment zone.

It works best to dry the corneal surface before placing the well to avoid slippage of the well. The patient is instructed to try not to blink and to continue looking straight ahead. With either method, the epithelium within the treatment zone needs to be completely covered with the dilute alcohol solution or there will be areas where the epithelium is more adherent. If there is a large amount of alcohol in the well, then a dry surgical spear can be used to remove the excess before lifting the well and rinsing copiously with balanced salt solution.

If the patient moves unexpectedly and the alcohol solution spills out of the treatment zone, then the eye should be quickly and thoroughly rinsed with balanced salt solution. In most cases, this

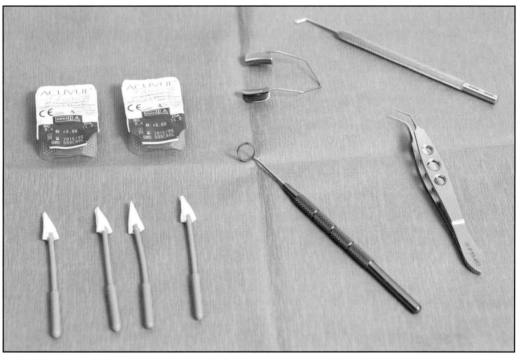

Figure 4-1. PRK uses a simple array of instruments, including a corneal well for dilute alcohol if needed and a standard hockey stick-type instrument for epithelial removal. (Photograph by Amanda Sneddon.)

may make the eye more injected or sore in the immediate postoperative period but will not affect the overall outcome. In these cases, it may be necessary to repeat the alcohol application to the treatment zone if it was not on long enough to break the bonds between epithelium and Bowman's membrane.

Once the well is lifted, the impression of the well is easily visible and a hockey stick-type blunt blade can be used to slide the epithelium off. It generally works best to sweep from peripheral to central in order to avoid a loose epithelium at the edge of the treatment zone. The instrument should always be angled in order to avoid unintentional incursion into the Bowman's membrane if the patient should move unexpectedly.

In some patients, the epithelium is particularly loose superiorly so care should always be taken in this location. Patients with known map-dot-fingerprint-type changes or corneal scars should also be approached cautiously as the epithelium may be loose over these areas.

There is variability between patients as to how adherent the epithelium is. In some cases, the epithelium can be swept off with a very smooth edge along the treatment zone. In other cases, the epithelium may be more adherent and more pressure might be needed to sweep it off. It is helpful to try to make the treatment zone edge as smooth as possible. Jagged or loose edges can lead to significant discomfort in the immediate postoperative period. During the epithelial removal, attention should be paid to corneal hydration. Once the contact lens is in place, it should be inspected at the operating microscope and any folded edges should be corrected in order to improve comfort for the first few days following PRK.

The advantages of alcohol-assisted epithelial removal are less discomfort for the patient as compared to the epikeratome at the time of surgery, the ability to control the epithelial removal zone by using a well of a specific diameter, and low cost (Table 4-2). This method can be used for patients with corneal scars and for retreatments following prior corneal refractive surgery as PRK or RK but should be avoided following LASIK as it may shift the flap.

TABLE 4-2. PHOTOREFRACTIVE KERATECTOMY WITH DILUTE ALCOHOL

ADVANTAGES	DISADVANTAGES
Less discomfort intraoperatively	Possibly longer recovery compared to epi-LASIK
Corneal scar not a contraindication	May lead to large or persistent fusion pattern
Low risk of intraoperative complication	Discomfort if alcohol spills outside of treatment zone
Simple technique and low cost	
Suitable for retreatment following prior corneal surgery	

The disadvantages are the possible increase in discomfort due to the use of alcohol and a longer recovery of visual clarity following contact lens removal in patients who have a large or persistent fusion line.

Photorefractive Keratectomy With Corneal Brush

The Amoils brush (Innovative Excimer Solutions Inc, Toronto, Canada) was introduced by Percy Amoils in 1995. It is a modified electronic toothbrush with a rotating brush size. It causes minimal discomfort for the patient and avoids the use of a blade. The epithelium can be removed quickly in order to preserve corneal hydration.

When using the corneal brush, the corneal surface is marked prior to epithelial removal to delineate the intended treatment zone. The brush tip should be moistened with a balanced salt solution prior to application to the cornea and should be remoistened each time. It is helpful to let the patient hear the brush before using it on the eye in order to avoid a startled patient. To avoid residual central epithelium, a circular motion is recommended while using the brush. Some surgeons keep a 9-mm marker on the eye in order to stabilize and guide the brush while using the brush in the center.

Electron microscope studies indicate that the brush leaves a smoother edge as compared to a blade alone and that it is comparable to the alcohol-assisted method. It is also a suitable technique for retreatment following previous corneal refractive surgery (Table 4-3).

The disadvantages are that, in some cases, residual epithelium may have to be removed with another instrument and eye movement can result in off-center epithelial débridement, which may require widening on one side. Irregularity of the epithelium at the edge of the treatment zone can lead to more discomfort and there has been discussion in the literature about the crushing effect of the brush, which may lead to a release of inflammatory cytokines. The disposable brushes will also increase the cost of the procedure.

LASEK

The technique of LASEK was developed to combine the advantages of flap creation in terms of speed of vision recovery and less discomfort with the safety of PRK. Several investigators have described variations of techniques.[2-5]

Most LASEK techniques involve using a dilute alcohol solution, which is contained in a corneal well in order to avoid spillage and possible damage to the limbal cells. Dilute alcohol cleaves the

TABLE 4-3. PHOTOREFRACTIVE KERATECTOMY WITH CORNEAL BRUSH	
ADVANTAGES	DISADVANTAGES
Minimal discomfort intraoperatively	Possible decentered débridement
Smooth edges of treatment zone	May need to remove residual epithelium with blade
Suitable for retreatment after prior corneal refractive surgery	May cause more discomfort due to release of inflammatory cytokines from crushed cells
Low risk of intraoperative complication	Slightly higher expense for disposables compared to alcohol-assisted PRK

TABLE 4-4. LASEK	
ADVANTAGES	DISADVANTAGES
Possibly less postoperative pain	Possible epithelial flap damage
Possibly increased recovery speed	More involved technique compared to PRK

epithelial cells from the basement membrane and allows separation of the epithelial sheet from the underlying Bowman's membrane. The alcohol is reabsorbed using a dry sponge and the corneal surface is rinsed with balanced salt or methylcellulose.

The epithelial sheet is then reflected back or rolled using sponges or a spatula to expose the treatment zone. Following laser ablation, the epithelial sheet is replaced and the bandage contact lens is placed. Variations of LASEK techniques include lifting the flap by injecting methylcellulose liquid under the flap using a cannula or creating a paracentral linear epithelial defect and reflecting the flaps in a butterfly pattern.

Advantages of LASEK may include less postoperative pain and faster visual recovery. Disadvantages include a slightly more complex technique and a possible epithelial flap shift or flap tear that would necessitate discarding the flap.

There has been some debate about whether replacing the epithelial flap has any beneficial effects in terms of decreased postoperative pain, speed of visual recovery, or reduced corneal haze. Some recent studies have shown there is no difference whether the epithelial flap is discarded or replaced.[5] Some surgeons routinely remove the epithelial flap (Table 4-4).

EPI-LASIK

Epi-LASIK was developed as a tool for creating an epithelial flap for LASEK without the use of dilute alcohol, which was thought to devitalize the cells. The epikeratome is a microkeratome device with a suction ring that uses an oscillating separator to cleave the epithelial cells (Figure 4-2). There has been debate about whether replacing the epithelial flap affords advantages over discarding the flap and most studies indicate the outcomes are equal regardless of flap removal or replacement.[6] There have been some small studies that indicate that replacement of the flap may slow recovery or lead to increased discomfort in the early postoperative period.

Many surgeons use the epikeratome and discard the flap in order to avoid the use of dilute alcohol and also to create a very smooth epithelial edge along the treatment zone. A smoother edge

Figure 4-2. Epi-LASIK involves an automated oscillating epikeratome separator that uses a vacuum suction ring to stabilize the cornea during the keratome pass. (Photographed by Amanda Sneddon.)

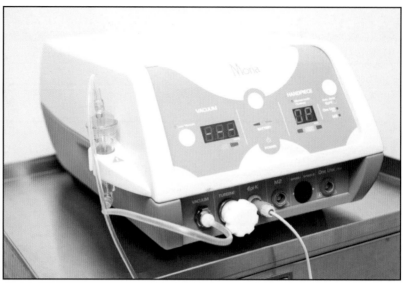

TABLE 4-5. EPI-LASIK	
ADVANTAGES	**DISADVANTAGES**
Faster vision recovery	More discomfort on the day of surgery
Small fusion line	Not suitable for retreatment after corneal surgery or cases with corneal scars
Smooth edge to treatment zone	Slightly higher risk of irregular astigmatism
	Slightly higher expense for disposables compared to alcohol-assisted PRK

without epithelial tags will generally lead to less discomfort in the first few days following surgery. Using the epikeratome allows for a more reliable ability to create that smooth edge as compared to PRK. Some surgeons also believe the epikeratome is superior to the corneal brush because it does not crush and disrupt the epithelial cells. There is evidence that when cells are crushed, they release inflammatory cytokines that will increase pain and possibly increase the risk of haze postoperatively.

The other advantage seen with epi-LASIK is a smaller fusion line in most cases when the epithelial healing reaches the center. This is likely a result of the smooth epithelial edge created by the epikeratome. With PRK, there is often a stellate fusion line that can lead to persistent ghosting for days to weeks after contact lens removal. More often with epi-LASIK, the fusion line is smaller and linear, leading to faster resolution of visual symptoms (Table 4-5).

Similar to the microkeratome in LASIK, the epikeratome uses a suction ring, which will lead to more discomfort for the patient for about 30 seconds during the treatment (Figure 4-3). Patients will experience pressure on the eye, the vision will dim or black out, and they will have a vibrating sensation during that time. If the lids are tight or the patient is squeezing, he or she will often feel pressure or a pinching sensation on the lids.

Allowing patients to hear the device in action prior to surgery can help them know what to expect, although the majority of patients will flinch involuntarily just as the pass is started after suction is on. By simply supporting the epikeratome and not holding it, the device will move with the patient and in most cases there is no loss of suction.

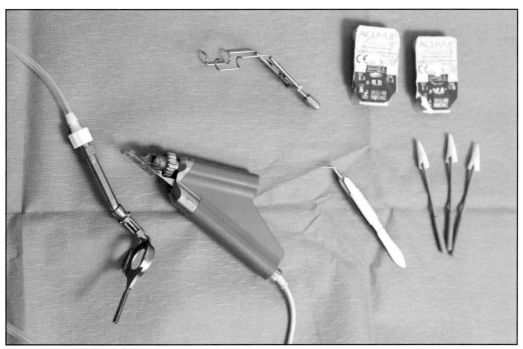

Figure 4-3. Epi-LASIK uses a suction ring and epikeratome (pictured above). Patients will experience about 30 seconds of pressure and the vision may dim out during the epikeratome pass for epi-LASIK. (Photograph by Amanda Sneddon.)

During surgery, the epikeratome does add some risk of irregular astigmatism if the separator tracks incorrectly. The separator follows Bowman's membrane so any scarring or disruption of Bowman's, such as map-dot-fingerprint, will be a contraindication to epi-LASIK. Retreatment following previous corneal refractive surgery should not be performed with the epikeratome.

TRANSEPITHELIAL PHOTOREFRACTIVE KERATECTOMY

Transepithelial PRK differs from PTK in that the beam profile is designed for epithelial removal for refractive PRK. This method has been reported over the years but has not been as widely used as mechanical methods of epithelium removal in the past due to the difficulty in accurately removing the epithelium with the excimer laser. Recent reports with the Schwind and Nidek lasers report results that are equal to the alcohol method of epithelial removal.[7,8]

With the transepithelial PRK (also called trans-PRK or T-PRK), recent studies report the epithelium and stroma are ablated in a single step using a transepithelial PRK nomogram. Dr. Luger reports a technique where refraction correction is done on the epithelial surface followed by phototherapeutic keratectomy to remove 55 μm in the center and 65 μm in the periphery of the cornea. For accurate transepithelial ablation, the difference in epithelial thickness between the center and the periphery of the cornea must be taken into account.

Advantages of transepithelial PRK include the simplicity of using the excimer laser for both the epithelial removal and the refractive stromal ablation and very smooth edges on the ablation zone (Table 4-6). Disadvantages may include more discomfort according to some studies.[9] Accuracy might be affected by humidity, as the epithelial thickness may vary with hydration.

TABLE 4-6. TRANSEPITHELIAL PHOTOREFRACTIVE KERATECTOMY	
ADVANTAGES	**DISADVANTAGES**
Simplicity of technique	Accuracy may be affected by humidity
Suitable for retreatment following prior corneal surgery	Proper nomogram required to account for differences in epithelial thickness from central to periphery

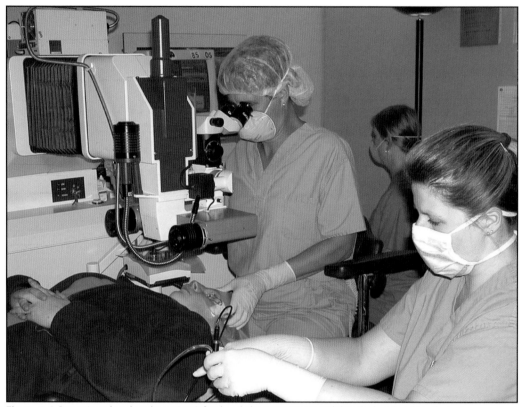

Figure 4-4. By resting a hand on the patient's forehead, the surgeon can stabilize the head and can feel when a patient may be restless or tense. (Reprinted with permission of Rick W. Triebwasser, BSc, COMT from Gimbel HV, Penno EE. *LASIK Complications: Prevention and Management*. 3rd ed. Thorofare, NJ: SLACK Incorporated; 2004.)

VOCAL-LOCAL (INTRAOPERATIVE COMMUNICATION)

During the past decades, a move toward topical anesthesia has revolutionized cataract surgery. In order to successfully perform any type of ophthalmic surgery with topical anesthetic, the patient must be able to cooperate and remain relatively still during the procedure. The concept of "vocal-local" has been talked about over the years and involves communicating with the patient as the surgery progresses. Talking the patient through the procedure, outlining the expected sights and sounds, and reassuring the patient during the process will allay anxiety and prevent startling.

Keeping a hand on the patient's forehead is a helpful technique that allows for stabilizing and guarding against unexpected head movement (Figure 4-4). In many cases, the surgeon can feel if the patient is about to cough or if the patient is feeling unwell and becomes restless before any sudden movements occur. This allows for a pause and a verbal check with the patient in order to make adjustments for the patient to be more comfortable for the remainder of the surgery.

POSTOPERATIVE SLIT-LAMP EXAM

A postoperative slit-lamp exam will ensure that the contact lenses are in place after the patient has been in recovery and that there are no foreign bodies, such as a lash under the contact lens. Occasionally, the contact needs to be repositioned or replaced. This postoperative slit-lamp exam gives the surgeon the opportunity to reinforce any specific instructions that the surgeon may feel are needed.

It can be helpful to have the patient's family member or companion sit in at the postoperative examination in order to help the patient remember any additional instructions. This examination only takes a matter of minutes and is reassuring to the patient that the contact is in place before he or she is discharged.

FUTURE

The increasing interest in surface ablation will drive advances in patient screening, pain management, and acceleration of vision recovery. Research will drive improvements in ablation profiles with the goal of reducing higher-order aberrations and improving vision quality. Continued advancements in prevention and treatment of corneal haze are also likely.

Regardless of the rapid evolution of corneal flap technology, surface ablation will continue to be a significant percentage of refractive surgeries performed for the foreseeable future.

SUMMARY

Epithelial removal techniques are the hallmark of surface ablation. Each technique has the potential for benefits or complications. An understanding of both surgical methods and epithelial healing is essential to optimizing results. Small refinements in technique, such as ensuring that no epithelial tags remain following alcohol-assisted PRK, can make a noticeable difference in postoperative comfort and vision recovery. Familiarity with all the epithelial removal techniques allows the surgeon to select the methods that work best for him or her to provide superior results and the fastest recovery following surface ablation.

REFERENCES

1. Sadaka A, Cherfan DG, Melki SA. Inadvertent LASIK flap creation over a soft contact lens. *J Refract Surg.* 2012;28(1):74-76.
2. Shah S, Sebai Sarhan AR, Doyle SJ, Pillai CT, Dua HS. The epithelial flap for photorefractive keratectomy. *Br J Ophthalmol.* 2001;85(4):393-396.
3. Taneri S, Zieske JD, Azar DT. Evolution, techniques, clinical outcomes and pathophysiology of LASEK: review of the literature. *Surv Ophthalmol.* 2004;49(6):576-602.
4. Camellin M. Laser epithelial keratomileusis for myopia. *J Refract Surg.* 2003;19(6):666-670.
5. Vinciguerra P, Camesasca FI, Randazzo A. One-year results of butterfly laser epithelial keratomileusis. *J Refract Surg.* 2003;19(2 suppl):S223-S226.
6. Taneri S, Oehler S, Koch J, Azar D. Effect of repositioning or discarding the epithelial flap in laser-assisted subepithelial keratectomy and epithelial laser in situ keratomileusis. *J Cataract Refract Surg.* 2011;37(10):1832-1846.
7. Luger MH, Ewering T, Arba-Mosquera S. Consecutive myopia correction with transepithelial versus alcohol-assisted photorefractive keratectomy in contralateral eyes: one-year results. *J Cataract Refract Surg.* 2012;38(8):1414-1423.
8. Buzzonetti L, Petrocelli G, Laborante A, et al. A new transepithelial phototherapeutic keratectomy mode using the NIDEK CXIII excimer laser. *J Refract Surg.* 2009;25(1 suppl):S122-124.
9. Kanitkar KD, Camp J, Humble H, Shen DJ, Wang MX. Pain after epithelial removal by ethanol-assisted mechanical versus transepithelial excimer laser debridement. *J Refract Surg.* 2000;16(5):519-522.

Techniques for Faster Recovery After Photorefractive Keratectomy

Daniel S. Durrie, MD and Theodore A. Pasquali, MD

Surface ablation has faced 3 issues that have prevented it from becoming the preferred laser refractive procedure: pain, haze, and slow visual recovery. Advances have improved methods, reducing pain and haze to manageable levels; however, the speed of visual recovery has continued to lag. If visual recovery could be shortened and brought to a speed equal to or even faster than LASIK, then, except in special cases, the need for the creation of a corneal flap would be eliminated, eliminating with it the risks and safety concern, albeit small, associated with corneal flaps. Laser refractive surgery would become more efficient without the need for all the resources (training, space, equipment, supplies, and personnel) that we currently dedicate to flap creation, and may also have biomechanical advantages. Additionally, the slower visual recovery has real-world consequences for the patient: at 1 week, some patients may not have legal driving vision. Improving the speed of visual recovery will have a meaningful impact on productivity, days off of work, social interactions, the ability to perform daily activities, and other areas related to quality of life.

Bandage contact lenses and improved excimer ablation profiles have modestly improved the speed of visual recovery but their benefits in this area have more or less plateaued. Otherwise, there has been generally little success in addressing the issue of faster visual recovery.

One technology that demonstrates promise is the Nexis ocular shield (NexisVision, Menlo Park, CA) (Figure 4A-1). It is a shield placed over the cornea at the end of surgery that provides visual recovery within the first hour after surgery, significantly faster than LASIK procedures, by optimizing the optics of the corneal surface during healing. We performed a prospective study of 55 eyes (28 patients) treated with PRK and placement of the Nexis shield and compared these patients to historical controls. Early data have shown equal if not superior visual recovery at day 1 compared to previously published data with sub-Bowman's keratomileusis (SBK)[1] and clear superiority to traditional PRK (Figure 4A-2). All shield patients demonstrated legal driving vision at day 1. Monocular vision results at days 3 and 7 (Figures 4A-3 and 4A-4) are roughly equal between the shield and SBK, with PRK demonstrating minimal improvement. There is a small decline in vision demonstrated at day 3 after removal of the shield, likely secondary to the transition from the optics of the shield to the re-epithelialized cornea. This has resolved by week 1 and during the first week, the best-corrected vision remains 20/20 or better at every visit (Figure 4A-5).

Additionally, the shield serves as a scaffold for corneal healing, speeding re-epithelialization of the cornea. While 85% of shield eyes took the usual amount of time to epithelialize as bandage contact lens eyes (3 days), 10% demonstrated epithelialization by day 2, and only 5% required a longer period to epithelialize. Not only does epithelialization appear to be faster in shield eyes, but it is also of superior quality (Figure 4A-6) when compared to the use of a bandage contact lens. This topographic quality has a demonstrable impact on vision: even though standard PRK eyes have re-epithelialized by week 1, the visual recovery continues to lag while 100% of shield eyes are 20/40 or better.

The shield is still in early development and is not widely commercially available. Comfort with the present design is not better than bandage lenses and this is a goal of future development. If this innovation can overcome the challenges, it would be transformative for surface ablation, providing superior visual recovery, faster epithelialization, and improved patient satisfaction.

Reference

1.   Slade SG, Durrie DS, Binder PS. A prospective, contralateral eye study comparing thin-flap LASIK (sub-Bowman keratomileusis) with photorefractive keratectomy. *Ophthalmology.* 2009;116(6):1075-1082.

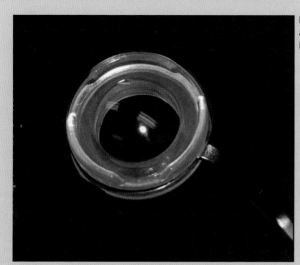

Figure 4A-1. The Nexis ocular shield atop applicator. (Reprinted with permission from NexisVision.)

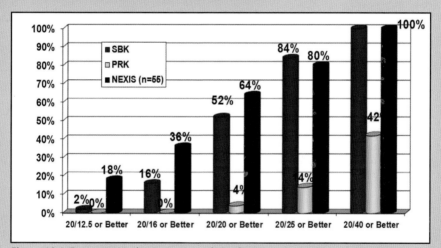

Figure 4A-2. Postoperative day 1 uncorrected visual acuity.

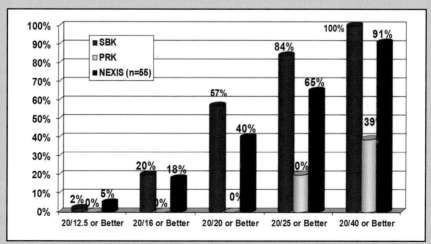

Figure 4A-3. Postoperative day 3 uncorrected visual acuity.

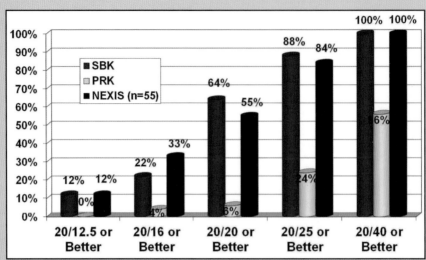

Figure 4A-4. Postoperative day 7 (week 1) uncorrected visual acuity.

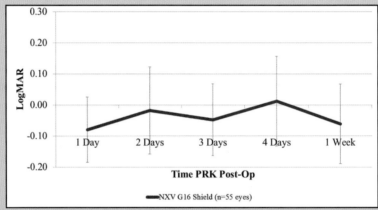

Figure 4A-5. Best-corrected visual acuity measurements at each visit for the Nexis shield.

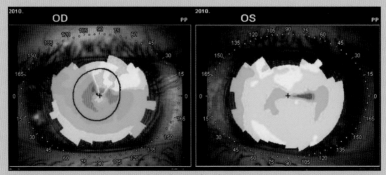

Figure 4A-6. Corneal topography 1 hour after bandage contact lens removal (ocular dexter) versus 1 hour after Nexis shield removal (oculus sinister) demonstrating greater corneal regularity and smoothness in the shield eye. (Reprinted with permission from NexisVision.)

Phototherapeutic Keratectomy

Phototherapeutic keratectomy (PTK) is a distinct treatment from refractive surface ablation. As indicated by the name, the intention of PTK is to treat corneal surface disorders, in contrast to photorefractive keratectomy (PRK), which is intended for the primary purpose of refractive correction (Table 5-1). PTK will typically use a beam profile with a zone size selected to suit a specific case.

The ablation is equal across the treatment zone and surgeons take advantage of this by using smoothing fluid to fill in low points, thereby ablating only elevated corneal lesions. PTK beam profile characteristics are also an advantage in transepithelial PTK techniques in which the epithelium will act as the masking agent, allowing for ablation of elevated areas where the epithelium is thinnest before breaking through over the low points.

PTK may be done to improve best-corrected acuities, such as in the case of corneal scarring. In other cases, it may be done to improve comfort, such as in cases of recurrent erosion or bullous keratopathy. In rare cases, it may be done for treatment of infection. Studies indicate that the smoother surface resulting from PTK can improve ocular surface health.[1]

PTK was approved in 1995 for the treatment of anterior corneal pathology to improve best-corrected visual acuity (BCVA) and for the treatment of symptoms, such as pain or foreign-body sensation. In the early years of excimer laser surgery, central islands were a more common indication for PTK. With advances in ablation profiles, central islands are rare at present time. Since Federal Drug Administration approval, treatment with PTK has been reported for a large variety of corneal conditions (Table 5-2).

Overall reported successful outcomes following PTK vary from greater than 50% to 95% of patients measuring improved BCVA.[2] However, a major drawback continues to be hyperopic shifts, which can range from +3 to +9 D following PTK.

PHOTOTHERAPEUTIC KERATECTOMY PATIENT SELECTION

Indications for PTK include raised lesions, such as Salzmann's nodular degeneration, stromal scars, including anterior corneal dystrophies and band keratopathy, and recurrent erosion. Surgeons have also used PTK smoothing following refractive ablation and for treatment of

Anderson Penno EE. *Surface Ablation:
Techniques for Optimum Results (pp 67-75).*
© 2013 SLACK Incorporated.

TABLE 5-1. INDICATIONS FOR PHOTOTHERAPEUTIC KERATECTOMY

DISORDER	EXAMPLE
Raised corneal lesions	Salzmann's nodular dystrophy
Anterior stromal scars	Anterior stromal dystrophy, band keratopathy
	Recurrent erosion
Irregular astigmatism	Following LASIK flap complications
Infectious keratitis	Acanthamoeba, fungal

TABLE 5-2. CONDITIONS TREATED WITH PHOTOTHERAPEUTIC KERATECTOMY

- Amyloidosis
- Anterior basement membrane dystrophy
- Avellino dystrophy
- Band keratopathy
- Bullous keratopathy
- Climatic droplet keratopathy
- Corneal scars after bacterial keratitis, epikeratophakia, herpes simplex keratitis, pterygium, radial keratotomy, trachoma, trauma, and vernal/atopic
- Viral infection (other)
- Fuchs' dystrophy
- Granular dystrophy
- Infectious keratitis including fungal and acanthamoeba
- Keratoconus nodules
- Lattice dystrophy
- Macular dystrophy
- Meesmann's dystrophy
- Recurrent erosion
- Reis-Bucklers dystrophy
- Salzmann's nodular degeneration
- Schnyder's crystalline dystrophy
- Stevens-Johnson syndrome
- Thygeson's superficial punctate keratopathy

TABLE 5-3. RECURRENCE FOLLOWING PHOTOTHERAPEUTIC KERATECTOMY

• Reis-Bücklers dystrophy	• Herpes simplex
• Macular dystrophy	• Recurrent erosion
• Epidemic keratoconjunctivitis	

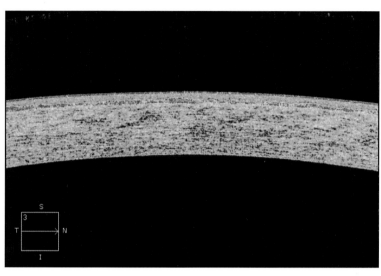

Figure 5-1. Corneal OCT may be helpful in surgical planning.

laser-assisted in situ keratomileusis (LASIK) flap complications, such as buttonhole. PTK has been used in the management of infectious keratitis, including fungal and acanthamoeba keratitis.

In some cases, the primary corneal disorder may recur (Table 5-3). Reis-Bücklers dystrophy and macular dystrophy have been reported to recur following PTK. Reactivation of the virus has been reported after PTK treatment for scarring from epidemic keratoconjunctivitis and herpes simplex keratitis. Recurrent erosion can recur at the edge of the treatment zone.

Systemic collagen vascular diseases, diabetes, or neurotrophic cornea may raise the risk of slow re-epithelialization or corneal melt. Ocular surface disease, such as dry eye and meibomian dysfunction, should be addressed. Exposure due to lid anomalies, which may be present in trauma, should be addressed prior to PTK treatment.

A thorough preoperative work-up should include slit-lamp, dilated examination, topography, pachymetry, and refraction, if possible. Additional testing such as a B-scan in trauma cases to rule out posterior segment pathology may be necessary.

Patient expectations should also be appropriate in terms of visual and refractive outcomes. For example, recurrent erosion can often be managed with topical treatment and the use of PTK may alter the refraction as a side effect of treatment. As noted above, significant hyperopic shifts can be a side effect of PTK.

SURGICAL PLANNING

Optical coherence tomography (OCT) may be useful in determining the depth of pathology (Figure 5-1). Topography can also be helpful in surgical planning and some surgeons have reported good results combining topography-guided ablation with PTK.[3] Ultrasound biomicroscopy has been discussed in the literature and may overestimate pathology.

TABLE 5-4. PHOTOTHERAPEUTIC KERATECTOMY SURGICAL PLANNING	
• Pathology	• Progressive/nonprogressive
• Depth	• Risk of recurrence
• Location	• Refractive effects
• Symptoms	

In contrast to refractive surface ablation, there are a wide variety of corneal conditions that may be considered for PTK treatment. The location, size, and depth of the corneal disease process may determine if PTK is a suitable option (Table 5-4). Very deep stromal opacities may not be amenable to PTK. Infectious conditions and some corneal dystrophies may be more likely to recur after PTK.

Refractive Effects of Phototherapeutic Keratectomy

Central PTK will have a hyperopic refractive effect proportional to the amount of stromal tissue ablated. The Munnerlyn formula is not as useful for PTK due to a number of factors. Diseased, scarred, or calcified corneal tissue will ablate at different rates than normal corneal stroma. In addition, the ablation may have weaker effects in the peripheral cornea due to oblique incidence of the beam profile. In some cases, peripheral debris may play a role in reduced peripheral ablation rates.[4]

While hyperopia is common with central PTK, induced astigmatism or myopia could result depending on the zone and location of PTK application. These effects must be taken into consideration for preoperative surgical planning. Hyperopic PRK ablation following PTK can be used to offset the refractive effects of PTK.

Depending on the ablation rates of the affected tissue, transepithelial PTK may provide a smoothing effect or may result in irregular astigmatism. Techniques to improve smoothing will vary depending on the corneal pathology and may include partial epithelial débridement, transepithelial ablation, the use of smoothing fluids, and mechanical scraping of elevated lesions.

In general, a larger ablation zone diameter will result in a smaller amount of induced hyperopia as predicted by the Munnerlyn formula. Peripheral blend zones can be used as well. Another general concept is that the cornea does not need to be completely clear in order to improve BCVA. The goal is to remove the least amount of tissue possible in order to improve BCVA.

Intended Outcome

With deeper treatments, the uncorrected acuity may be worse due to induced refractive error with the goal of improving the best-corrected acuity. In other cases, PTK may be a temporizing measure to delay corneal transplant or lamellar graft. The goal for some treatments may be the reduction of pain, such as in bullous keratopathy or recurrent corneal erosion. In all cases, the patient should have an appropriate understanding as to the goals of treatment, possible complications, and alternatives to PTK in order to make an informed choice about whether to undergo PTK treatment.

Ablation Rates

The targeted ablation depth should be determined preoperatively based on slit-lamp examination, topography, and other measurements, such as OCT. Ablation rates will vary depending on the corneal disorder and techniques. Calcified lesions may have a lower ablation rate than corneal stroma and corneal scars may ablate more quickly than healthy stromal tissue. Masking fluids may also have ablation rates that may vary, and masking fluids will typically be reapplied throughout treatment.

For lengthy treatments, corneal dehydration may influence ablation rates. Increased corneal dehydration can lead to more rapid ablation and should be taken into consideration for complex treatments.

Thin Corneas

PTK is generally recommended for disorders that affect the anterior one-third of the cornea. Recommendations include leaving a residual bed thickness of 250 μm or more and for not ablating more than 33% of the corneal tissue when treating with PTK. Consideration for the location of treatment and underlying pathology will be necessary for each case. For example, a scar due to corneal ulcer may be located at the thinnest area of the cornea.

The advent of corneal cross-linking is already impacting treatment recommendations for PTK in conditions such as keratoconus. There has been discussion of corneal cross-linking in cases of infectious keratitis and postrefractive surgery ectasia. It seems likely that cross-linking will be applied to a wider variety of cases in the future.

PHOTOTHERAPEUTIC KERATECTOMY TECHNIQUES

The techniques of PTK will vary from case to case. Most cases will be done using topical anesthetic and a mild sedative, such as a benzodiazepine. For cases that are not using the epithelium for masking, the epithelium is removed using a hockey stick with or without the use of dilute alcohol. The patient will be instructed to look at the fixation light for central ablations, and the surgeon will need to position the patient's head or eye if the intended treatment zone is off center.

A masking solution, such as dextran 0.1% or hydroxymethylcellulose 0.7% to 2%, can be spread onto the cornea in a smooth layer in order to mask low areas and expose high corneal irregularities for ablation. Masking fluid should be reapplied intermittently throughout the PTK ablation with care to avoid too much fluid. Most central PTK ablations for stromal opacities are done with a 6- to 7-mm zone.

Elevated lesions that are not amenable to mechanical débridement may be treated by local débridement of the elevated lesion followed by a 1- to 2-mm ablation to reduce the height of the lesion. This can be followed by a larger 4- to 5-mm zone or the use of masking agents to produce a smoothing effect.

Some surgeons advocate examination at the slit-lamp at three-quarters of the planned ablation depth in order to avoid overablation. It is not necessary in most cases for the cornea to be completely clear in cases of corneal opacities (Figure 5-2). Consideration should be given to the residual corneal bed thickness and to the ablation rate of scars or of calcification in band keratopathy, which may differ from normal stroma.

Recurrent erosions that do not respond to medical management can be treated with PTK. Loose epithelium should be débrided followed by PTK to cover the area of erosion to a depth of 5 or 6 μm. Recurrent erosions can continue at the edges of the PTK treatment zone if treatment does not cover the entire area. Induced astigmatism may occur depending on location and depth of treatment.

Figure 5-2. Scheimpflug imaging can be useful for assessing pachymetry.

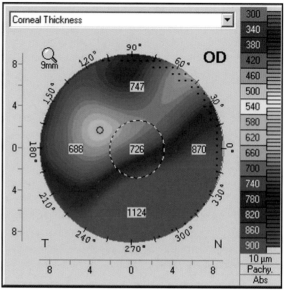

MECHANICAL DÉBRIDEMENT BEFORE PHOTOTHERAPEUTIC KERATECTOMY

Some surgeons use a combined technique of débridement with a blade followed by PTK for elevated lesions such as Salzmann's nodules. A combination of manual excision of fibrotic scar with PTK has also been described for retreatment following radial keratotomy (RK). For recurrent corneal erosion, the techniques include débridement of all loose epithelium followed by PTK across the entire visual axis in order to avoid irregular astigmatism.

TRANSEPITHELIAL PHOTOTHERAPEUTIC KERATECTOMY

This technique takes advantage of the features of epithelial thickness in irregular corneal surfaces. The epithelium is thinner over elevated areas and thickest in the lower areas. Due to this fact, the PTK ablation will break through preferentially over the corneal elevations, and the epithelium will protect the lower areas until the entire ablation reaches that level. Another feature of epithelium is that it produces blue fluorescence during excimer ablation. This allows the surgeon to visually track the areas of epithelial ablation and stromal ablation to determine the ablation endpoint.

Ashrafzadeh and Steinert described a standardized technique for PTK treatment of flap striae following LASIK.[5] An important part of this technique is the combination of trans-epithelial PTK with masking fluid. They describe using transepithelial PTK to ablate the raised striae just until breakthrough begins to appear in the valleys between the striae. They then describe using the masking fluid to protect the low areas to allow for further ablation of the peaks. In this way, a smoother corneal surface is produced.

Trans-epithelial PTK has been used for corneal scars following epidemic keratoconjunctivitis, for treatment of irregularity due to flap striae and buttonholes following LASIK, and for treatment following RK.

MITOMYCIN C AFTER PHOTOTHERAPEUTIC KERATECTOMY

Mitomycin C can be used following PTK in order to prevent haze formation. The decision to use mitomycin C may be based on the etiology of the corneal disorder, ablation depth, and laser platform used. Mitomycin C in concentrations ranging from 0.002% to 0.02% placed on the treatment zone for 20 sec and up to 2 min following PTK ablation has been reported.

The use of PTK with mitomycin C has been described in Salzmann's, treatment of scars following epidemic keratoconjunctivitis, and haze resulting from PRK over RK. Mitomycin C use has been widely reported and is considered safe as a one-time application treatment on the corneal surface within the treatment zone. There have been reports of permanent corneal edema following PTK for basement membrane dystrophy followed by repeat mitomycin C drops over 6 days.[6]

Mitomycin C may be less effective if there is active inflammation at the time of treatment.

PHOTOTHERAPEUTIC KERATECTOMY AND CORNEAL CROSS-LINKING

There have been increasing reports of combining PRK or PTK with corneal cross-linking. The Athens procedure described by Kanellopoulos and colleagues combines PTK, topography-guided PRK, and corneal cross-linking for treatment of keratoconus.[7]

PTK with a 6.5-mm zone to 50 μm is performed first to remove the epithelium. This is followed by topography-guided partial PRK with mitomycin C 0.02% for 20 sec following PRK. Only a partial refractive treatment is performed with the intent to reduce refractive error but to limit ablation depth. A 5.5-mm optical zone is used to target steepening next to the cone. Finally, corneal cross-linking is performed.

A substantial number of patients have a favorable outcome in terms of vision and stability; however, some patients will go on to have worsening ectasia or in some cases visual acuity that is worse than prior to treatment. Complications include delayed epithelial healing and haze.

Although keratoconus and thin corneas are considered to be contraindications to corneal excimer ablation, the rationale in this approach is that if a patient is likely to need a corneal transplant, then it is possible to avoid transplant with combined treatment. According to Kannellopoulos, removal of the corneal epithelium and Bowman's layer with PTK will allow better penetration of ultraviolet-A light into the stroma. In addition, the use of topography-guided PRK will provide a more regular corneal shape, which may have more biomechanical strength to withstand IOP fluctuations or eye rubbing.

PHOTOTHERAPEUTIC KERATECTOMY COMBINED WITH OTHER SURGICAL TECHNIQUES

PTK can be combined with other surgeries like amniotic membrane grafts and penetrating keratoplasty (Table 5-5). PTK prior to cataract surgery can improve visual outcome and refractive accuracy for patients with anterior corneal opacities. Following pterygium removal or LASIK flap complications, PTK has been used for treatment of irregular astigmatism.

TABLE 5-5. COMBINED PHOTOTHERAPEUTIC KERATECTOMY

- Before or after penetrating keratoplasty (PKP)
- Following pterygium removal
- After complicated LASIK flap
- Combined with amniotic membrane graft
- Before cataract or refractive surgery
- Combined with corneal cross-linking

PHOTOTHERAPEUTIC KERATECTOMY FOLLOWING FEMTOSECOND LASER FOR RECURRENT EROSION

Recently, a series of cases have been reported of PTK for recurrent erosion following femtosecond laser LASIK for treatment of myopia.[8] They reported that transient diffuse lamellar keratitis and mild haze developed following PTK over a femtosecond flap but that final BCVA was unaffected.

PHOTOTHERAPEUTIC KERATECTOMY IN THE DEVELOPING WORLD

A series of 203 eyes were reported in a retrospective study at a tertiary care center in the developing world.[9] Many of these patients were from Northern India and the most common diagnosis was bullous keratopathy following cataract extraction. Salzmann's nodular degeneration and spheroidal degeneration were the next most common indications for PTK. Due to poor socioeconomic conditions and lack of donor corneas, PTK provides the best alternative available for pain reduction and improved vision.

PHOTOTHERAPEUTIC KERATECTOMY COMPLICATIONS

There are complications following PTK that can occur following any type of surface ablation (Table 5-6). These included delayed epithelial healing, corneal haze, and infection. Ectasia and perforation have also been reported following PTK, highlighting the need to consider PTK ablation depth and preoperative pachymetry. Complications specific to PTK include recurrent corneal disease, which is possible in specific cases as noted earlier.

McCally and colleagues reported a differential haze response in a rabbit model in which 2 different rabbits treated with an identical PTK protocol developed different haze responses.[10] They measured haze response with a scatterometer and with confocal microscopy. Following PTK, the haze response did not necessarily correlate with paired eyes such that fellow eyes of one rabbit responded differently in some cases. They could not correlate findings in this study with speed of re-epithelialization and haze did not correlate with the PTK treatment session.

These findings indicate that haze formation is more complex than simply ablation depth or speed of defect closure. It may be even more difficult to predict haze response in PTK treatment of abnormal corneas. As noted above, mitomycin C may be less effective in the prevention of haze in corneas with active inflammation.

TABLE 5-6. PHOTOTHERAPEUTIC KERATECTOMY COMPLICATIONS

• Delayed re-epithelialization	• Recurrent corneal disease
• Corneal haze	• Ectasia
• Infection	• Perforation
• Reactivation of herpes simplex	

SUMMARY

There are a number of different corneal disorders involving the anterior cornea that can be treated using PTK. The large variety of pathology that may be amenable to PTK has generated an equally large array of techniques and combinations of techniques. PTK candidates will need an individualized treatment plan to suit their specific case.

REFERENCES

1. Dogru M, Katakami C, Miyashita M, et al. Ocular surface changes after excimer laser phototherapeutic keratectomy. *Ophthalmology.* 2000;107(6):1144-1152.
2. Rapuano CJ. Excimer laser phototherapeutic keratectomy in eyes with anterior corneal dystrophies: preoperative and postoperative ultrasound biomicroscopic examination and short-term clinical outcomes with and without an antihyperopia treatment. *Trans Am Ophthalmol Soc.* 2003;101:365-394.
3. Vinciguerra P, Camesasca FI. Custom phototherapeutic keratectomy with intraoperative topography. *J Cataract Refract Surg.* 2004;20(5):S555-563.
4. Ginis HS, Katsanasaki VJ, Pallikaris IG. Influence of ablation parameters on refractive changes after phototherapeutic keratectomy. *J Refract Surg.* 2003;19(4):1-6.
5. Ashrafzadeh A, Steinert RF. Results of phototherapeutic keratectomy in the management of flap striae after LASIK before and after developing a standardized protocol: long-term follow-up of an expanded patient population. *Ophthalmology.* 2007;114(6):1118-1123.
6. Pfister RR. Permanent corneal edema resulting from the treatment of PTK corneal haze with mitomycin: a case report. *Cornea.* 2004;23(7):744-747.
7. Kanellopoulos AJ. Comparison of sequential vs same-day simultaneous collagen cross-linking and topography-guided PRK for treatment of keratoconus. *J Refract Surg.* 2009;25(9):S812-S818.
8. Kremer I. Recurrent corneal erosion following uneventful IntraLASIK treated by phototherapeutic keratectomy. *Eur J Ophthalmol.* 2012;22(suppl 7):120-125.
9. Sharma N, Prakash G, Sinha R, Tandon R, Titiyal JS, Vajpayee RB. Indications and outcomes of phototherapeutic keratectomy in the developing world. *Cornea.* 2008;27(1):44-49.
10. McCally RL, Connolly PL, Stark WL, Jain S, Azar DT. Identical excimer laser PTK treatments in rabbits result in two distinct haze responses. *Invest Ophthalmol Vis Sci.* 2006;47(10):4288-4294.

Laser Ablation
Standard, Topography-Guided, Wavefront-Optimized, Wavefront-Guided

Following epithelial removal, refractive surface ablation will require some method of excimer laser ablation. With newer lasers, there are wider choices for the refractive surgeon (Table 6-1). These include the increasingly popular wavefront and wavefront-guided treatments (Figure 6-1).

When photorefractive keratectomy (PRK) was first introduced, there were 3 categories of excimer lasers based on the beam delivery: broad-beam, scanning-slit, and flying spot. Over the following decades, excimer lasers have advanced with software and shutters to allow for a sophisticated delivery of excimer laser energy with precision that has allowed for the development of customized wavefront treatments. Features such as variable repetition rate have been included for some platforms to reduce the thermal impact of treatment.

Refractive surgeons must be familiar with the characteristics of the laser in use at their surgery center. Lasers will differ in terms of beam delivery, software versions, and hardware versions, such as the availability of eye trackers and cyclotorsion control. Variability in algorithms, availability and accuracy of wavefront treatments, and tendency to produce corneal haze should also be understood when planning surface ablation using a specific excimer laser. It is also essential to control the humidity and temperature in the laser suite in order to have consistently accurate results.

PHOTOABLATION

Excimer is a term to describe the excited dimer, which is created by mixtures of gases that emit energy when they return to the resting state. All commercially available excimer lasers use an argon fluoride halogen mix that emits ultraviolet light with a 193-nm wavelength (Figure 6-2). As described in Chapter 1, it was originally intended for industrial use but was found to produce precise effects on biologic tissue.

Photoablation involves evaporation of the surface tissue without transmission to the tissue below. This feature allows for surface modifications in the form of refractive correction without damage to the underlying stroma.

Initially, commercially available lasers used a fixed broad beam. Over time, the scanning slit was employed with a rectangular pattern that moves over the cornea in a linear or rotating pattern as well as the flying spot, which uses a small-diameter spot to produce a more accurate ablation

Anderson Penno EE. *Surface Ablation: Techniques for Optimum Results (pp 77-87).*
© 2013 SLACK Incorporated.

TABLE 6-1. TYPES OF ABLATION PROFILES

• Standard (conventional)	• Wavefront-guided
• Topography-guided	• Phototherapeutic keratectomy
• Wavefront-optimized	

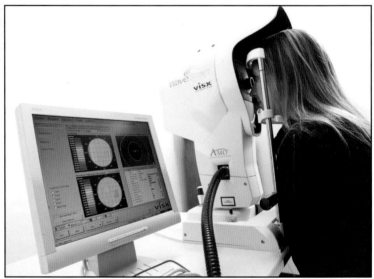

Figure 6-1. The latest generation of lasers include some that have the capacity for wavefront-guided ablation profiles with iris recognition and cyclotorsion adjustment. (Photograph by Amanda Sneddon.)

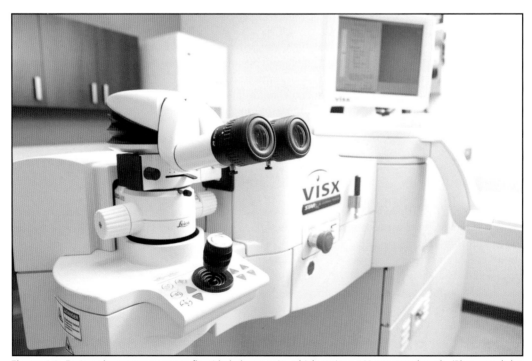

Figure 6-2. Excimer lasers use an argon fluoride halogen mix, which emits a 193-nm wavelength. (Photograph by Amanda Sneddon.)

Munnerlyn Formula: $\mathbf{T = (Dh^2)/3}$

T = thickness in microns

D = power in diopters

h = optical zone diameter in mm

Figure 6-3. The Munnerlyn formula describes the relationship between ablation depth and refractive result. This formula is not as predictive for PTK or advanced wavefront ablations.

pattern. Modifications over the years have included shutters to provide a variable spot size with broad-beam lasers, along with variable repetition rates.

The Munnerlyn formula describes the relationship between the ablation depth and the refractive result (Figure 6-3). As ablation patterns become more complex, this formula may underestimate the amount of tissue ablated due to the additional corrections of higher-order aberrations. As noted in Chapter 5, the ablation rates of abnormal corneas, smoothing solutions, and calcified lesions will vary.

VISUAL ACUITY VERSUS VISUAL FUNCTIONING

Visual acuity as measured by the Snellen chart gives limited information regarding visual functioning, yet is the most widely reported outcome for refractive surgery. A variety of other measures can be done, including field testing, color vision, contrast sensitivity, and glare testing; however, Snellen acuity remains the most practical method for routine in-office testing from visit to visit. The clinician generally relies on subjective satisfaction to determine if further testing is warranted.

In cases of symptomatic vision disturbances, refraction, topography, and wavefront mapping can be helpful along with slit-lamp and funduscopic examination. Mesopic functioning is more sensitive to variations of higher-order aberrations likely in part due to larger pupil diameter. In very small pupils, diffraction will be the limiting factor. For this reason, the superiority of wavefront treatment as compared to standard ablation may be less for patients with very small pupils.

NEURAL LIMITS

Due to the size of the photoreceptor mosaic, the ability to correctly discern objects is limited to between 20/8 and 20/10. Resolution of objects smaller than this limit can result in a phenomenon called aliasing in which the object is detected but is not interpreted correctly (Figure 6-4). When aliasing occurs, the object may appear to have a different shape than it actually does. This is also described in Chapter 2.

Neural limits mean that, regardless of the correction of higher-order aberrations, there will be a limit to the ability to provide "super vision" or acuity better than 20/10. There is some discussion regarding the effects of higher-order aberrations on depth perception. As discussed later in this chapter, some presbyopic ablation patterns include selective correction of higher-order aberrations in order to provide more depth of focus.

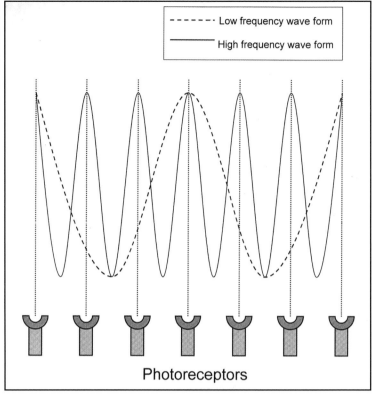

Figure 6-4. Aliasing occurs when the frequency of an image is smaller than the neural limit and is interpreted as a different shape as a result. (Reprinted with permission from Gimbel HV, Penno EE. *LASIK Complications: Prevention and Management.* 3rd ed. Thorofare, NJ: SLACK Incorporated; 2004.)

NEURAL ADAPTATION

In addition to the impact of ablation patterns, higher-order aberrations, age, pupil size, and other factors on visual functioning, neural adaptation can play a larger role in patient satisfaction. It is clear that patients will respond differently to a multifocal intraocular lens (IOL), monovision, and other types of vision correction. For example, many patients will adjust easily to progressive lenses in spectacles, whereas others may feel nauseated and off balance with progressives and will never adapt to that type of correction.

Unfortunately, it can be difficult to predict a patient's ability for neural adaptation to a specific type of correction. When possible, it is helpful to trial alternatives, such as monovision with contact lenses under a variety of conditions prior to correcting surgically. It is more difficult and in many cases not possible to trial multifocal patterns for IOL correction; the surgeon must rely on history of the patient to decide if he or she may be a good candidate. Historical factors, such as chronic difficulty with glasses prescriptions, might indicate poor ability to adapt to alternative vision correction methods.

STANDARD ABLATION

For several years after the introduction of the excimer laser, the refractive ablation profiles were designed to correct the sphere and the cylinder with a blend zone in the periphery. This basic correction would be analogous to a spectacle correction. In the early years, there was some variation between laser platforms regarding optical zones and transition zones.

```
Treatment Information (Spectacle Plane) ─────────────────
Procedure:                Myopia and Astigmatism
Desired Correction:         -6.25 DS   -0.50 DC x 171°    12.50 mm
Physician Has Specified a Surface PRK Treatment


Laser Information (Corneal Plane) ──────────────────────
Total Ablation Depth:        77 µm
```

Figure 6-5. Wavefront treatments will remove more tissue than standard ablation. The same correction as noted previously will remove 95 µm with wavefront-guided ablation, almost 24% more tissue.

Over time, there were reports regarding higher-order aberrations, coma and spherical aberration in particular, that are increased with standard ablation profiles. This increase in higher-order aberrations can impact visual functioning, particularly in low light. Larger pupil size and higher corrections will increase the likelihood of increased higher-order aberrations that may impact visual functioning.

Standard ablation, also called conventional ablation, has more recently been largely replaced in many surgery centers by ablations based on wavefront theory. This change is an effort to reduce the possible higher-order aberrations that may be induced using a standard ablation profile. Wavefront treatments will remove more tissue than a standard ablation (Figure 6-5).

TOPOGRAPHY-GUIDED ABLATION

Topography-guided ablation uses preoperative manifest refraction for refractive correction, and treatment of higher-order aberrations and adjustment of asphericity are based on corneal topography. Studies indicate that topography-guided ablation offers accurate results for primary refractive surgery.

There are also many reports in the literature supporting the use of topography-guided ablation for irregular astigmatism following laser-assisted in situ keratomileusis (LASIK) or corneal transplant and for treatment of keratoconus. Recently, surgeons have reported success in using the "Athens Protocol" where cross-linking and topography-guided surface ablation are performed simultaneously rather than sequentially.

WAVEFRONT-GUIDED ABLATION

As described in Chapter 2, an aberrometer is used to measure the higher-order aberrations and the refraction using infrared light and this information is used for wavefront-guided ablations. Surgeon input is necessary in order to adjust for chromatic aberration due to the wavelength used for aberration measurements, which will measure approximately 0.50 D less myopic than the manifest refraction with accommodation relaxed. Refractions generated by the aberrometer can be influenced by accommodation and this should be taken into consideration when selecting the measurements for treatment as well as in formulating a treatment plan.

The most common wavefront analyzers use the Hartmann-Shack method, which uses a grid of microlenses to measure the reflected infrared light (Figure 6-6). The reflected rays are compared to an ideal wavefront model to create the aberration map. Other methods include the Tscherning method, which projects a grid onto the cornea, and the resulting distortions are used to measure aberrations of the eye (Table 6-2). Another method that is used in the Nidek OPD-scan (Nidek Inc, Fremont, CA) is dynamic skiascopy, which measures the refraction of the eye over 1440 points. This method may take a longer time to process data for acquisition but can simultaneously capture topography for closer alignment of topographic data with aberrometry.

Some surgeons will consider aberrometry when assessing dissatisfied patients. The root mean square (RMS) is a summation of higher-order aberrations but may not be correlated with clinical

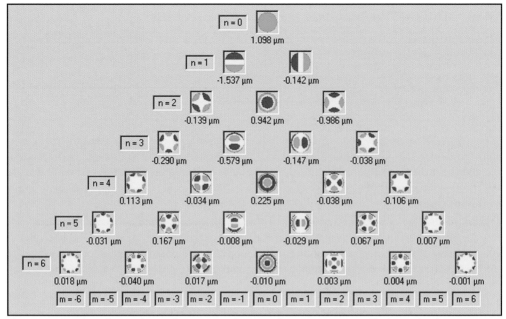

Figure 6-6. Zernike polynomials are often presented as a graphic representation of higher-order aberrations.

TABLE 6-2. ABERROMETER METHODOLOGY

- Hartmann-Shack: Uses a grid of micro-lenses to measure reflected infrared light for comparison to an ideal wavefront model.
- Tscherning method: Projects a grid onto the cornea and uses distortion of the grid to measure aberrations.
- Dynamic skiascopy: Measures the refraction of the eye over 1440 points.

symptoms. Another global measurement that can be generated from wavefront analysis is point spread function (PSF) (Figure 6-7). PSF will correlate with visual symptoms in some cases but is also affected by pupil size due to diffraction effects.

All of these measurements can be affected by ocular surface disease due to the powerful refractive effect of the tear film. In addition, wavefront aberrometry will be affected by all medial opacities, including early lens changes. Aberrometry provides a useful tool but must be considered in the context of clinical findings.

As discussed in Chapter 3, pupil size can be a factor when planning a wavefront treatment. Large pupils may be problematic for iris landmarking. Small pupils may not provide adequate wavefront data. Attention to lids and tear film is important as well (Figure 6-8). Dry eye or medial opacities can affect the data acquisition (Figures 6-9 and 6-10).

Debate about the superiority of wavefront-guided versus wavefront-optimized is ongoing in the literature.[1-3] There is some suggestion that wavefront-guided ablation may be superior to wavefront-optimized ablation with respect to postoperative higher-order aberrations and contrast sensitivity.

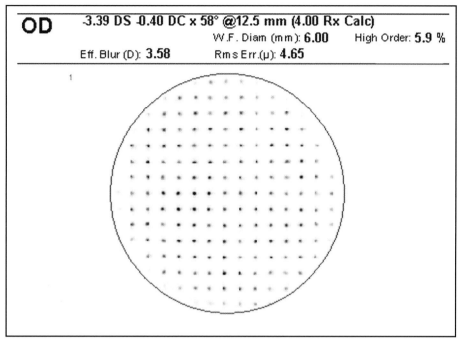

Figure 6-7. Hartmann-Shack is the most common method of aberration used at the present time.

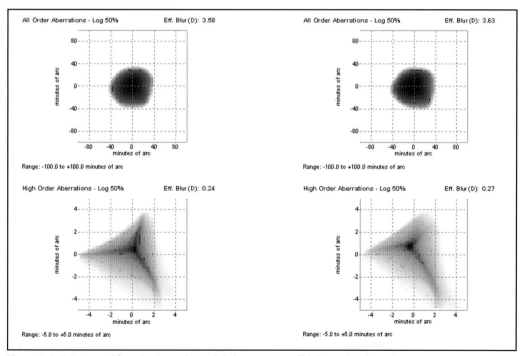

Figure 6-8. Point spread function is used as a global assessment of higher-order aberrations.

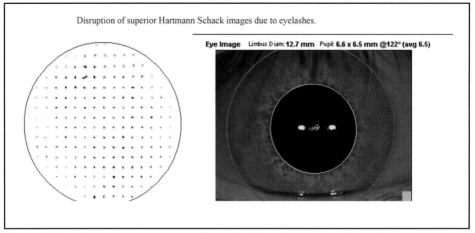

Disruption of superior Hartmann Schack images due to eyelashes.

Eye Image   Limbus Diam: 12.7 mm   Pupil: 6.6 x 6.5 mm @122° (avg 6.5)

Figure 6-9. Wavefront aberrometry can be affected by lid interference and other factors such as dry eye. (WaveScan system, Abbott Medical Optics Inc.)

Figure 6-10. Medial opacities can affect the quality of data collected on wavefront aberrometry.

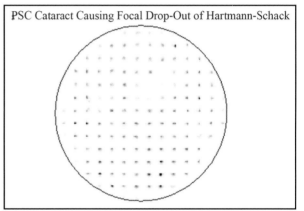

PSC Cataract Causing Focal Drop-Out of Hartmann-Schack

WAVEFRONT-OPTIMIZED

Wavefront-optimized treatments use wavefront theory to create an aspheric refractive ablation profile. This is also sometimes called "optimized aspheric" ablation. The natural corneal shape is aspheric with the curvature flattening in the periphery. The standard profiles with the blend or transition zone did not duplicate this asphericity and resulted in increased higher-order aberrations as noted previously. The efficacy of wavefront-optimized versus wavefront-guided ablation continues to be debated.

EYE TRACKING AND CYCLOTORSION CONTROL

Eye trackers have been incorporated into excimer lasers for many years. For older broad-beam and scanning-slit lasers, it was possible to center the treatment visually; however, eye trackers have always been required for the flying spot lasers as it is not possible to center the treatment by simply watching the ablation pattern.

All modern excimer lasers now use eye tracking. Eye tracking for x/y centration uses the pupil border to lock onto centration. Trackers will compensate for saccades and smaller head movements, such as mild drift in position. The laser will not fire once the pupil is out of range. In most cases, the surgeon will recognize that the pupil is moving out of range and will release the foot pedal before the laser stops firing.

Cyclotorsion is important for more complex ablation patterns or for high astigmatism correction. When a patient lies flat, a naturally occurring cyclotorsional reaction may occur such that the patient's eye could rotate up to 10 degrees or more. Head tilt can also cause a rotation when positioned under the laser. In an effort to adjust for this, surgeons can make a mark at 6 o'clock at the slit lamp using a needle to make a slight mark, which is filled in with a gentian marker. Then, when the patient is positioned under the laser, his or her head can be tilted to adjust the mark to the proper position.

A more sophisticated and accurate solution of iris recognition with cyclotorsional control has been added to some wavefront-guided excimer platforms. This technology allows for landmarking of the iris at the aberrometer and then provides real-time iris recognition and recognition with a rotational adjustment at the time of laser ablation. This technology can also account for centroid shifts of the pupil due to miosis. Cyclotorsion adjustments will enhance the accuracy of the wavefront ablation and also improve accuracy of astigmatic treatments.

ABLATION DEPTH

Different ablation patterns will remove different amounts of tissue. The Munnerlyn formula has been used to calculate ablation depth and can be used to estimate ablation depths for standard treatments. The formula calculates depth of the ablation (in micrometers) equal to the square of the diameter of the optical ablation zone measured in millimeters multiplied by the diopters of correction divided by 3.

More complex treatments, such as wavefront-guided ablations, will use more tissue than a conventional treatment. In order to offset this effect, laser manufacturers have developed tissue-sparing algorithms, which some manufacturers state will remove 20% to 30% less tissue.

There is discussion in the literature regarding the depth of ablation as a risk factor and, as ablation patterns become more sophisticated, they are removing more tissue. Some surgeons will consider using mitomycin C for an ablation depth greater than 75 µm or greater than 6 D of myopia.

ABLATION TYPE

Haze may be more common with different laser platforms and surgeons should become familiar with their particular laser in order to decide when to use prophylactic mitomycin C (Table 6-3). There have been studies on older lasers to indicate that the risk of haze was higher with broad-beam lasers as compared to flying-spot lasers.[4] The variability of reports about when to use mitomycin C in surface ablation is likely due to these differences between laser systems, refractive techniques, and risk of haze. There is likely variability between patient physiology and haze occurrence as well.

There are no large studies to compare commercially available lasers using a standard surface ablation technique with modern excimer technology. In general, visually significant haze is uncommon. During the past decades, there have been significant changes to laser ablation patterns, including larger treatment zone, variable repetition rates, and variable spot sizes on some laser platforms. These advances may provide a smoother ablation surface and may reduce heat generation, which are factors that may impact the risk of corneal haze following surface ablation.

Vinciguerra has published reports on using smoothing fluid intraoperatively in order to provide the smoothest surface possible in order to optimize results.[5] However, as discussed in Chapter 5, the risk factors for corneal haze following excimer laser ablation are not well understood.

TABLE 6-3. POSSIBLE RISK FACTORS FOR CORNEAL HAZE

- Small treatment zone
- Ablation depth
- Hyperopic correction
- High myopic correction
- Laser platform type: ablation profile, potential heat generation
- Pre-existing pathology (in PTK)
- Patient physiology
- Exposure to ultraviolet light
- Pregnancy following laser ablation

MITOMYCIN C

Mitomycin C is an antimetabolite that has been used in concentrations ranging from 0.002% to 0.02% placed on the treatment zone for 20 seconds and up to 2 minutes for prevention of corneal haze following primary refractive PRK and PTK. Haze may develop in spite of mitomycin C, so patients at risk should be followed postoperatively and should be started on topical steroid in order to prevent visually significant haze.

Some surgeons feel mitomycin C is only needed in very high corrections, and others use it for all cases above a certain correction or ablation depth. There is a wide range of opinions regarding when to use mitomycin C and the specifics of the application concentration and duration. When considering the use of mitomycin C, it may be helpful for surgeons to look at studies specific to their laser system and to discuss results with other users of that specific system.

CORNEAL COOLING

As noted above, there has been discussion about corneal haze and the role of heat generation intraoperatively. Haze generation is related to inflammation and postoperative ice packs have been recommended for comfort but it is possible that cooling postoperatively as well may also reduce generation of haze.

Intraoperatively, corneal cooling techniques include the use of a frozen surgical spear, which is placed on the corneal surface for approximately 30 seconds following laser ablations. Some surgeons will use a larger volume of chilled balanced salt solution to rinse the cornea following ablation.

PRESBYOPIC ABLATION

Multifocal biaspheric ablations have recently been developed for treatment of ametropia and presbyopia.[6] This is also being investigated with the femtosecond laser.[7] There are recent reports of a biaspheric pattern and of selective treatment of higher-order aberrations in order to improve near vision in presbyopic patients.[6,8]

These presbyopic patterns are reported to have satisfactory results; however, it is not clear yet if this may become a common alternative option to monovision or reading glasses for presbyopic surface ablation candidates. An advantage to monovision is that it is straightforward to trial in a contact lens to determine if the patient will tolerate this type of correction. The selection of patients for presbyopic surface ablation may be more difficult if there are patients who are unable to tolerate this type of ablation pattern. More studies will be needed that include patient satisfaction as an outcome measure to determine if this will become a more common procedure for presbyopic patients.

SUMMARY

At present, there is not a clear consensus as to the superiority of wavefront-guided versus wavefront-optimized ablation, but most surgeons are moving away from standard ablations to these more advanced options. Topography-guided ablation is reported for use in primary refractive corrections but is more widely reported for treatment of irregular astigmatism, such as keratoconus.

Due to the number of excimer platforms, a variety of treatment options, including surface ablation or flap-based treatment and variability in the patient population (age, correction, pupil size, ocular surface disease), studies do not show a consistently superior result for any of these advanced ablation profiles at this time.

REFERENCES

1. Moshirfar M, Betts BS, Churgin DS, et al. A prospective, randomized, fellow eye comparison of WaveLight® Allegretto Wave® Eye-Q versus VISX CustomVue™ STAR S4 IR™ in laser in situ keratomileusis (LASIK): analysis of visual outcomes and higher order aberrations. *Clin Ophthalmol.* 2011;5:1339-1347.
2. Stonecipher KG, Kezirian GM. Wavefront-optimized versus wavefront-guided LASIK for myopic astigmatism with the ALLEGRETTO WAVE: three-month results of a prospective FDA trial. *J Refract Surg.* 2008;24(4):S424-S430.
3. Padmanabhan P, Mrochen M, Basuthkar S, Viswanathan D, Joseph R. Wavefront-guided versus wavefront-optimized laser in situ keratomileusis: contralateral comparative study. *J Cataract Refract Surg.* 2008;34(3):389-397.
4. Pallikaris IG, Koufala KI, Siganos DS, et al. Photorefractive keratectomy with a small spot laser and tracker. *J Refract Surg.* 1999;15(2):137-144.
5. Vinciguerra P, Camesasca FI, Torres IM. Transition zone design and smoothing in custom laser-assisted subepithelial keratectomy. *J Cataract Refract Surg.* 2005;31(1):39.
6. Uthoff D, Polzl M, Hepper D, Holland D. A new method of cornea modulation with excimer laser for simultaneous correction of presbyopia and ametropia. *Graefes Arch Clin Exp Ophthalmol.* 2012;250(11):1649-1661
7. Peter M, Kammel R, Ackermann R, et al. Analysis of optical side-effects of fs-laser therapy in human presbyopic lens simulated with modified contact lenses. *Graefes Arch Clin Exp Ophthalmol.* 2012;250(12):1813-1825.
8. Khalifa MA, Allam WA, Khalifa AM. Improving near vision in presbyopic eyes by selective treatment of high-order aberrations. *Clin Ophthalmol.* 2011;5:1525-1530.

7

Early Postoperative Care

Early postoperative care includes from the day of surgery until the contact lens is removed and the patient is in the legal range for driving. This can vary from 3 days to 1 week depending on the patient and on the procedure.

First 24 Hours

Most patients will take a sedative such as Ativan (Pfizer, New York, NY) 1 to 2 mg sublingual for surgery. It is a good idea to have the patient rest in a recliner for a few minutes following surgery to be sure he or she is not feeling faint. In rare cases, even a low dose of benzodiazepine can cause balance problems, so patients should be warned of this possible side effect. Patients should be reminded not to drink alcohol following the sedative.

Before the patient leaves the surgery center, he or she should be accompanied by a friend or relative and should be checked at the slit-lamp to ensure the contacts are in position and that there are no foreign bodies, such as a lash or fiber under the contact. Occasionally, the contact may need to be removed and replaced. Taking the time to do this just after surgery is worthwhile. If the foreign body is discovered a day or 2 postoperatively, then the removal and replacement of the contact can result in a shift of the new epithelium, which can result in delayed healing and more discomfort.

The immediate postoperative check will take only a few minutes and is an opportunity to remind the patient that the comfort will worsen as the freezing drops wear off, the vision will worsen over the first few days, and the 2 eyes can heal differently (Figure 7-1). If the patient has a close friend or relative in attendance, it is helpful to have him or her listen to the instructions in order to help the patient remember postoperative instructions.

Encourage patients to limit visually demanding activities, use frequent gentle ice packs with eyes closed, and use preservative-free artificial tears to improve comfort. Prepare the patient for the worsening of vision and comfort that is likely to occur over the next few days (Table 7-1). For most people, the comfort and vision will tend to worsen after 24 to 48 hours before improving. A follow-up phone call the evening after surgery will calm the patient and allow him or her to ask any questions he or she may have.

Most surgeons use a combination of fourth-generation fluoroquinolone, topical steroid, and a nonsteroidal anti-inflammatory until the epithelial defect is closed (Figure 7-2). Frequent

Anderson Penno EE. *Surface Ablation: Techniques for Optimum Results (pp 89-97).* © 2013 SLACK Incorporated.

Figure 7-1. A brief post-operative slit-lamp exam is useful to double-check that the contact is in good position and that there is no foreign body such as a lash under the contact lens. It is also an opportunity to review postoperative instructions with the patient and with his or her companions. (Photograph by Amanda Sneddon.)

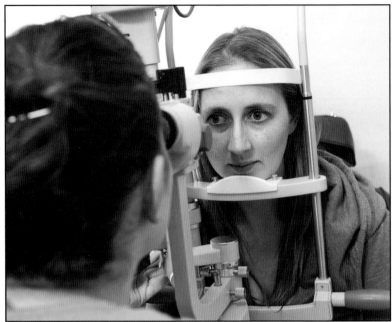

TABLE 7-1. WHAT TO EXPECT IN THE FIRST FEW DAYS FOLLOWING SURFACE ABLATION

- Worsening visual acuity over 24 to 72 hours
- Worsening comfort for the first 48 hours followed by improvement
- Photophobia
- Stinging
- Burning
- Foreign-body sensation
- Ghosting of vision
- Monocular diplopia
- Difficulty keeping eyes open

*Most patients will find the first 24 hours have only minor discomfort with worsening over the second 24 hours followed by improvement; vision may continue to worsen until re-epithelialization is complete.

preservative-free tears are often recommended as well. Often, an oral pain medication is provided, such as codeine. Patients can take a nonprescription analgesic such as acetaminophen or ibuprofen and, if started early and taken as directed for the first 48 hours, it may not be necessary to take a stronger pain medication. Depending on the oral pain medication prescribed, the patient should be educated as to whether he or she can safely combine it with an over-the-counter medication.

Topical tetracaine is usually provided for limited use. Patients can be instructed that it can be used if they wake up and cannot get back to sleep due to discomfort. If patients are comfortable inserting soft contacts, then they can use the tetracaine and insert a new bandage contact lens if the contact comes out.

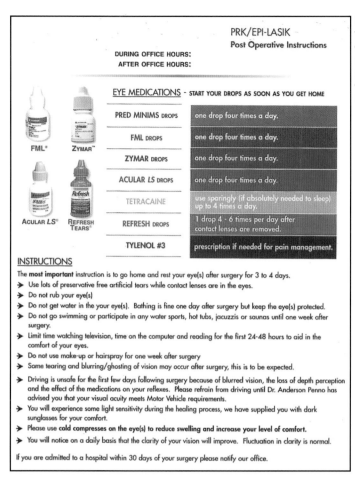

Figure 7-2. A patient instruction sheet with photographs of the topical medications can be helpful to patients in recognizing various medications prescribed. This will allow for better compliance with recommended drop regimens.

Advise patients that if they need to use the tetracaine, then they should take an oral analgesic if they have not taken one within the recommended interval, repeat an ice pack, and use preservative-free tears. When patients are informed that overuse of topical anesthetic may slow healing, most patients will not use it at all.

It is uncommon for the bandage contact lens to come out but a patient who is a contact lens wearer can be given a spare contact lens to insert if necessary. This would be a situation where the use of tetracaine might be necessary. Including a spare contact lens in the postoperative supplies will allow the patient who is comfortable handling contacts to manage a contact lens loss at home rather than necessitating an office visit.

A courtesy telephone call can be beneficial the evening after surgery. By scheduling an evening phone call with the on-call technician, the patient is assured he or she will have an opportunity to ask any questions he or she may have forgotten to ask while in the office. It also allows the technician to reassure the patient about what may be normal symptoms. This can avoid patient calls late at night. Excessive worry can increase patients' perception of discomfort and a calming telephone call can smooth the recovery.

24 TO 48 HOURS POSTOPERATIVELY

There is variation in follow-up routines depending on the surgeon. A slit-lamp exam within 1 or 2 days can help detect early infection or inflammation. While corneal infiltrates are uncommon,

TABLE 7-2. CAUSES FOR LOOSE EPITHELIUM

- Eye rubbing
- Contact lens loss
- Contact lens movement
- Removing the bandage contact too early

early detection allows for prompt treatment.[1] Due to the expected worsening of vision and comfort over the first 48 hours, it may not be possible to detect infection or infiltrates without inspection at the slit-lamp. Complications will be discussed in Chapter 10.

Many patients will report that it feels like something is under the contact lens. Early inspection at the slit-lamp will reassure the patient that there is nothing under the contact and that this sensation can be a normal part of healing. Photophobia is more common between 24 and 48 hours as the comfort is worsening.

Visual acuity on the first postoperative day will typically range from 20/25 to 20/60. There are some patients who are 20/20 on day 1 and, infrequently, vision can be as poor as 20/200. Higher corrections are more frequently followed by transient corneal edema, which usually clears when the epithelial defect is healed. These patients may have very poor vision in the 20/200 range in the first few days after surgery. Patients will often note that vision and comfort will vary between eyes, and they can be reassured that these differences in healing between eyes are common and do not predict final vision outcome.

Uncommonly, the contact lens may shift and cause shifted epithelium under the contact lens (Table 7-2). If it is a small area of shifted epithelium, then the contact can be left in place, although it is likely that the patient will be more uncomfortable. In many cases, removing and replacing the contact will lead to a larger area of shifted epithelium so, if at all possible, it is best to leave the contacts in place until the defect is healed.

POSTOPERATIVE DAYS 3 TO 5

The range of time for the epithelial defect to heal will typically range from 3 to 5 days with the majority of patients able to have the bandage contact lenses removed on day 4. Healing time is similar between different types of contact lenses.[2,3] The timing of the postoperative visits may vary between surgeons and, provided the patient's symptoms are progressing as expected, it is not necessary to see the patient every day. For example, the patient may be seen on day 1 and then again on day 4.

Between appointments is another opportunity to schedule a telephone call (Table 7-3). For example, if the patient is seen on day 1, then a call can be scheduled on postoperative day 2. In general, calling the patient later in the day on the second postoperative day can be useful as by that time, most patients will be over the peak of the most significant discomfort and while the vision will likely still be quite blurry, the comfort should be improving. Again, this allows for reassurance about the most expected symptoms as well as reminders about drop regimens and follow-up plans.

A sample schedule would be as follows: a phone call in the evening after surgery, slit-lamp examination on day 1, phone call in the evening on day 2, and slit-lamp exam on day 4 for contact lens removal. These proactive calls will result in happier, calmer patients and will reduce calls to the on-call system or office.

There is overlap in healing between patients due to differences in epithelial removal technique, degree of correction, and use of mitomycin C. In rare cases, it may take a full week for the

TABLE 7-3. SCHEDULE OF TELEPHONE CALLS

- Day 1: Evening call to confirm correct medication use and answer questions.

- Day 3: Patients will have an opportunity to discuss any issues at postoperative day 1 appointment and will generally not return until day 4 or 5. This interim appointment is an opportunity to reassure patients, if necessary, as the vision may be worsening at this point.

- Day 6: For some patients, a call the day after the contact lens is removed can provide reassurance as there will likely continue to be some visual disturbances relating to tear film and to the fusion line.

epithelium to heal. All patients undergoing surface ablation should be counseled that it is not possible to predict healing and that there may be additional visits needed in the first few days after surgery.

Care should be taken to make sure the epithelium is completely healed with a visible fusion line before taking the bandage contact lens out. If there is a visible defect or if there is an obvious loose epithelium, then the contact lens should be left in for an additional day. Taking the contact lens off too early can result in sloughing of the epithelium, which will necessitate replacing the contact and delaying the healing. In some cases, the contact can be removed in one eye earlier than the fellow eye.

Once the epithelial defect is healed, the antibiotic and nonsteroidal antibiotic drops can be stopped. Most surgeons will continue a topical steroid 4 times daily for a month and then will be on a tapering dose over the next weeks to months. Many patients will have uncorrected vision in the legal range for driving when the contacts are removed. If patients are legal to drive, then the next visit may not have to be for 3 to 4 weeks. Patients who are not legal to drive when the contacts are removed should be monitored within a week in order to document when they are within the driving limit.

DRIVING ABILITY

Legal requirements for driving vision may vary depending on jurisdiction. Legal to drive standards are not 20/20, so patients should be cautioned that they may choose to wait a few days before driving and they may need to avoid night driving to start. Going somewhere as a passenger at night before driving will allow patients to decide if they are comfortable enough to drive at night.

It is important for patients to understand before undergoing surgery the exact time when they will be legal to drive and will feel comfortable driving. Patients will often underestimate recovery time and will often be overscheduled on a regular basis with home and work obligations. Encourage patients to plan for alternate transportation for a week if possible following surgery.

Patients will be happier to be back to usual activities sooner than expected rather than to have unrealistic expectations about recovery. Patients may be legal to drive before the contacts are removed. It may be risky for patients to drive while bandage contacts are in place as a shift in the contact lens can cause them significant pain and tearing. For that reason, patients should be counseled not to drive until contacts are removed and vision is documented to be within legal standards. Many patients also will require documentation of uncorrected vision in order to update their driver's license.

TABLE 7-4. CAUSES FOR SLOW RECOVERY

- Slow re-epithelialization: Overuse of topical anesthetic, patient healing factors.
- Persistent fusion line: Large initial fusion line may form due to irregular epithelium at the edge of the treatment zone, loose epithelium, reabrasion.
- Persistent astigmatism: Undercorrection of astigmatism, persistent fusion line
- Dry eye: May be exacerbated by large fusion line, preoperative dry eye, and meibomian dysfunction.
- Hyperopia: Over-response in myopic corrections, under-response in hyperopic correction, larger than expected initial hyperopic shift, will be more problematic for presbyopic patients.

SLOW RECOVERY

Most patients will recover from surface ablation within the time frames expected but infrequently, there will be a delay in re-epithelialization in one or both eyes. There may also be a slow recovery of visual quality due to persistent or large fusion lines (Table 7-4). This can occur regardless of the epithelial removal method and without a complication such as reabrasion or shifted epithelium under the contact lens. In cases with mitomycin C, a slower-than-average re-epithelialization might be expected, and this delay can occur in cases without mitomycin C.[4]

In rare cases, it may take a week for the epithelium to heal. This will not necessarily have any long-term effects on final acuities. Patients can be reassured that while it can be frustrating, it will not impact the outcome. These cases will require additional visits every few days to monitor for infection and monitor the size of the defect. Using preservative-free drops where possible may help speed recovery.

Patients with a large or persistent fusion line will have more ghosting and more fluctuations of vision that may be present for a few to several weeks. In some cases, there will be induced astigmatism on refraction. Snellen acuity may overestimate functional acuity such that the patient reads the chart well but has significant quality of vision symptoms. For these patients, additional support may include documentation for additional time off or modified work duties and more frequent postoperative visits to provide reassurance. Frequent preservative-free tears or temporary punctal plugs might help; however, symptoms will typically resolve over time. A few patients may go on to need an enhancement but it is important to wait long enough to be sure that epithelial remodeling is complete, which may be up to 6 months.

ADVERSE REACTIONS TO MEDICATIONS

The most common adverse reaction can be nausea or vomiting from oral pain medication containing codeine. During the preoperative assessment and counseling, patients should be asked about sensitivities to medications that will be prescribed for use after surgery. Patients who have not used specific oral medications previously should be counseled as to possible side effects and should be advised to discontinue the medication and call if these develop.

Many surgeons offer a benzodiazepine, such as sublingual Ativan, on the day of surgery. In most cases, this is very well tolerated but in rare cases, patients may experience significant imbalance as a result. For patients who have taken a sedative, it is important to caution them after surgery to be aware of this potential side effect and to be particularly careful with stairs or, in Northern climates, icy sidewalks in winter.

Patients will be required to have a driver to take them home and a companion to watch for signs of imbalance to avoid a fall. Patients should also be advised not to drink alcohol after taking a sedative. Reactions to topical medications will be discussed in Chapter 10.

PREOPERATIVE KERATOMETRY AND REFRACTION

Patients should be provided with a copy of their preoperative keratometry and refraction for their records. Preoperative pachymetry is helpful in the case of later intraocular lens implant power calculations. Corneal power following surface ablation will not be measured correctly using standard keratometry and these preoperative measurements can be used for accurate intraocular lens calculations.

If these preoperative measurements are not available, then contact lens overrefraction can be used to determine corneal power. There are a number of other methods that have also been reported, including the Aramberri Double-K, the Latkany Flat-K, the Feiz and Mannis, the R-Factor, the Corneal Bypass, the Masket, the Haigis-L, and the Shammas postrefractive adjustment methods.[5]

SUMMARY

The early postoperative care of surface ablation patients is focused on pain management and surveillance for infection, which is fortunately rare. Scheduled telephone calls can be a benefit to both patients and staff to avoid patient anxiety and reduce calls to the on-call system.

REFERENCES

1. de Rojas V, Llovet F, Martínez M, et al. Infectious keratitis in 18,651 laser surface ablation procedures. *J Cataract Refract Surg.* 2011;37(10):1822-1831.
2. Grentzelos MA, Plainis S, Astyrakakis NI, et al. Efficacy of 2 types of silicone hydrogel bandage contact lenses after photorefractive keratectomy. *J Cataract Refract Surg.* 2009;35(12):2103-2108.
3. Edwards JD, Bower KS, Sediq DA, et al. Effects of lotrafilcon A and omafilcon A bandage contact lenses on visual outcomes after photorefractive keratectomy. *J Cataract Refract Surg.* 2008;34(8):1288-1294.
4. Kremer I, Ehrenberg M, Levinger S. Delayed epithelial healing following photorefractive keratectomy with mitomycin C treatment. *Acta Ophthalmol.* 2012;90(3):271-276.
5. McCarthy M, Gavanski GM, Paton KE, Holland SP. Intraocular lens power calculations after myopic laser refractive surgery: a comparison of methods in 173 eyes. *Ophthalmology.* 2011;118(5):940-944.

Advanced Surface Ablation

Richard J. Duffey, MD

Surface ablation, whether photorefractive keratectomy (PRK) or laser epithelial keratomileusis (LASEK), has become increasingly popular in mainstream laser vision correction in the United States. Surface ablation has increased from 15% of all laser vision correction cases in 2009 to the current level of 29% in the latest survey of US Trends in Refractive Surgery as reported by the membership of the International Society of Refractive Surgery subset of the American Academy of Ophthalmology in 2011.[1] A total of 167,000 PRK and LASEK cases were performed in 2011, up from 76,000 in 2009 in this same group of refractive surgeons. Most refer to modern surface ablation as advanced surface ablation, emphasizing improvements in technology (such as larger optical and blend zones, pupil and cyclotorsion tracking, high-order aberration identification and treatments), surgical techniques (such as perioperative ocular surface disease identification and treatment, use of mitomycin C, nonsteroidal anti-inflammatory agents, more potent steroids, vitamin C, and administration of cold balanced salt solution to decrease inflammation), and improved postoperative pain management.

There are myriad reasons for this increase in advanced surface ablation over laser-assisted in situ keratomileusis (LASIK), not the least of which is an increased conservatism among refractive surgeons to minimize the risk of keratectasia in a variety of corneas. The Randleman study[2] published in 2008 suggested more cautious guidelines for LASIK and surface ablation in some patients based upon several criteria: patient age less than 30 years, decreased central corneal thickness below 500 μm, presence of irregular anterior corneal topographical patterns (such as asymmetric bow-tie, skewed radial axis, and forme fruste keratoconus), degree of myopia exceeding -8.00 D, and a final residual stromal bed thickness below 300 μm. Although not all US ophthalmic surgeons may agree with these specific and exact guidelines,[3] these are becoming increasingly useful standards in borderline cases to help surgeons and patients sort out the safest options when considering laser vision correction.

There are numerous other circumstances where advanced surface ablation may be a superior alternative to LASIK. It has been my experience that very flat corneas (less than 40 D) are more difficult to applanate, to place a suction ring upon, and to center perfectly either with the femtosecond laser or modern microkeratomes. The same can be said in patients with very deep-set orbits and prominent brows. Previous LASIK patients undergoing retreatments years after the original procedure (especially when the original flap thickness is not known or cannot be measured or when the original flap was cut with a femtosecond laser) and postradial keratotomy patients are prime examples where surface PRK is on the increase as an alternative to LASIK. Likewise, patients who have epithelial issues, such as map-dot fingerprint dystrophy, may do better with PRK than LASIK due to the regeneration of a fresh, new, smooth epithelium following surface ablation.

Perhaps the most important aspect of laser vision correction, whether as advanced surface ablation or LASIK, is good communication between the patient and doctor with excellent informed consent. Given the longer healing period of surface ablation versus LASIK, patients must be made aware of the need for a curtailed work schedule in the first several days following surgery. These patients are often familiar with numerous friends and family members who have had laser vision correction, most commonly LASIK, so their expectations are geared for the rapid healing response of LASIK.

From a procedural standpoint, I prefer the Amoils brush (Innovative Excimer Solutions Inc, Toronto) for epithelial removal and the use of mitomycin C, 0.02%, as a 30-second application on all PRK patients, whether primary or secondary procedures. The Air Optix Night and Day high water content, high oxygen permeability bandage soft contact lens (Ciba Vision Corporation, Duluth, Georgia) is used typically for 5 days postoperatively along with a topical antibiotic and steroid 4 times a day for that first week. The antibiotic is discontinued upon completion of the epithelial healing and the removal of the bandage contact lens, but the fluorometholone topical steroid is used in a tapering fashion over an 8-week period.

I have found Ester-C (Inter-Cal, Prescott, AZ), 1000 mg per day for a minimum of 3 months, to be an excellent adjunct for healing and minimizing scar tissue formation. As an added advantage, many patients remain on Ester-C when they realize less susceptibility to viral colds and overall improved general health and well-being while taking it. Topical lubricants are imperative in the early, mid, and late postoperative period (often for 3 to 6 months), in a nonpreserved form as both a drop during the day and as a gel or ointment at night.

About one-third of my patients use acetaminophen with codeine or, very rarely, a stronger narcotic, Lortab (UCB Pharma, Brussels, Belgium), during the first several days following PRK surgery. Perhaps the greatest adjunct in that early postoperative period is the use of ice-cold compresses to minimize swelling of the eyelids and to improve the overall comfort of the patient. The old adage of "under-promise and over-deliver" certainly holds true for surface ablation given its slower healing rate relative to LASIK surgery.

I explain to patients that vision will decrease in the first several days and discomfort will increase during that same period of time, just the opposite of LASIK surgery. As such, they are not alarmed and expect this as a normal postoperative course. In my practice, I have found pregabalin, oral antidepressants, and oral anxiolytics to be of little help during the healing process. On the other hand, meticulous care of the ocular surface with omega-3 fish oils (taken orally as 2400 to 3000 mg per day for 3 to 6 months), punctal plugs, and occasionally Restasis eye drops can significantly reduce postoperative dry eye signs and symptoms, making the postoperative period more tolerable and speeding the healing process.

As always, an ounce of prevention is worth a pound of cure. Thus, treat dry eye and ocular surface disease such as blepharitis, meibomitis, trichiasis, and conjunctivitis before embarking on any laser vision correction, especially advanced surface ablation. Be aggressive in the early postoperative period to keep the ocular surface smooth, moist, and healthy to allow patients a rapid return of high-quality visual function and greater satisfaction with their choice of laser vision advanced surface ablation.

REFERENCES

1. Duffey RJ, Leaming D. Trends in refractive surgery in the United States: The 2011 ISRS/AAO Refractive Surgery Survey (abstract). *International Refractive Surgery: Science and Practice*, October, 2011.
2. Randleman JB, Woodward M, Lynn MJ, Stulting RD. Risk assessment for ectasia after corneal refractive surgery. *Ophthalmology*. 2008;115(1):37-50.
3. Duffey RJ, Hardten R, Lindstrom L, Probst LE. Ectasia after refractive surgery. *Ophthalmology*. 2008;115(10):1849.

8

Postoperative Care in the First 6 Months

With proper preoperative counseling, most patients will be prepared for the first days to few weeks following surface ablation. Most patients will also have an uncomplicated postoperative course over the next 6 months; however, there can be a wide range of experiences between patients. Some will have few concerns even if the vision is slow to recover, while others may remain anxious even with excellent Snellen acuity as the quality of vision and other factors, such as dry eye, may be improving. There is a wide range of healing responses within the first few months after surgery and often differences between fellow eyes.

1 to 6 Months Postoperatively

Topical Steroid Regimen

Many surgeons use a tapering dose of topical steroid over the first 4 months to reduce the risk of haze.[1] For example, some surgeons will advise fluorometholone (FML) 4 times daily for the first month, 3 times daily for the second month, twice daily for the third month, and once daily for the fourth month (Table 8-1). The potency of the steroid used may vary depending on the specifics of the patient and the specific laser used for treatment. Topical steroids may also help with dry eye symptoms within the first few months as the corneal nerves are recovering.

Preservative-free prednisolone can be used initially in order to avoid preservative effects on surface quality early in the recovery phase. For high corrections, the steroid may be tapered more slowly. If haze is identified at the postoperative slit-lamp examination, then the topical steroid may be held at the current dose or may be increased back to 4 times daily or more. For most cases, the standard taper can be followed.

Postoperative Examination Schedule

Postoperative visits approximately every 6 weeks while on a topical steroid will allow for intra-ocular pressure measurements to detect a steroid response (Table 8-2). These visits are also helpful in particular for reassuring patients who may be experiencing a slower-than-usual visual recovery

Anderson Penno EE. *Surface Ablation:*
Techniques for Optimum Results (pp 99-107).
© 2013 SLACK Incorporated.

TABLE 8-1. SAMPLE TOPICAL STEROID SCHEDULE

- Day 1 through re-epithelialization: preservative-free prednisolone QID
- 1st month: FML QID
- 2nd month: FML TID
- 3rd month: FML BID
- 4th month: FML QD

FML, fluorometholone; QID, 4 times a day; TID, 3 times a day; BID, twice a day; QD, once a day.

TABLE 8-2. SAMPLE POSTOPERATIVE VISIT SCHEDULE

- Day 1: Slit-lamp examination to check contact lens placement and rule out keratitis
- Day 4: Removal of bandage contact, uncorrected vision measurement
- 1 Week: If necessary to document legal to drive status (some patients will be legal to drive when the bandage lens is removed and will not need this visit)
- 1 Month: Uncorrected acuity, refraction, slit-lamp examination, IOP measurement
- 2.5 Months: Uncorrected acuity, refraction, slit-lamp examination, IOP measurement (if patient tapering off steroids, then next visit at 6 months, sooner if not)
- 6 Months: Uncorrected acuity, refraction, slit-lamp examination, IOP measurement, cycloplegic refraction, and mapping for patients considering enhancement

due to initial hyperopia or due to persistent fusion line. Persistent fusion line can cause ghosting and may also result in measured astigmatism that can take several weeks to resolve.

Common Postoperative Concerns

Presbyopic patients in particular can be troubled by the hyperopic shift that is often seen just after surface ablation. Patients often complain about computer work in particular. Young patients in computer-intensive occupations will also be more likely to experience fatigue or blurred vision early in the postoperative period.

Night vision is not often a chief complaint with the exception of patients with requirements for night driving, such as professional drivers or less commonly, night shift workers. In most cases, night vision will recover within a few weeks, but some people may need more time. Supporting the patient with work-related documentation for additional time off or for a temporary work modification is sometimes necessary.

Dry eye can also be a frequent complaint in the first few months.[2] Encouraging a daily routine with warm compresses twice daily and frequent artificial tears can help the patient manage dry eye symptoms. The use of preservative-free tears may be helpful in the first few weeks or if the patient continues to use tears very frequently.

Treatment of coexisting conditions, such as blepharitis or allergies, can improve patient comfort and may improve clarity of vision by improving the tear film. In the first few months, temporary punctal plugs may be helpful and, for persistent dry eye after 3 to 6 months, permanent plugs or cyclosporine A drops may be necessary.

Within the first weeks to months following surface ablation, epithelial remodelling will cause a shift in refraction ideally from mild hyperopia to plano. Sharpness of vision, dry eye, and night vision will also improve. Some patients will measure persistent astigmatism due to the fusion line. Understanding these healing patterns will help the refractive surgeon reassure and manage postoperative surface ablation patients.

In most cases, if a patient is at increased risk for these side effects, it can be predicted from the preoperative assessment and preoperative counseling should include a discussion about what to expect with an emphasis on specific issues. For example, if a patient wears eyeglasses full-time, then it is likely he or she will be more prone to dryness as a result of more exposure once he or she no longer wears glasses.

People in specific occupations, such as paramedics, may be more sensitive to initial difficulties due to low light because of the variety of conditions under which they may have to drive and do visually demanding tasks, such as starting intravenous lines. Careful attention to these details along with specific preoperative counseling will allow for a smoother postoperative course.

For most patients, it is also helpful to consistently counsel them that improvements in acuity might occur for up to 6 months and that the 2 eyes may sharpen up at different rates. Setting proper expectations for enhancement is also important. Often, patients will be comparing the 2 eyes by closing or covering one eye. Emphasizing binocular functioning may help in patient adjustment to minor differences between fellow eyes.

REFRACTIVE INSTABILITY WITHIN THE FIRST 6 MONTHS

A mild hyperopic shift is often measured in the first few months following surface ablation. Hyperopia will be particularly troubling to presbyopes and near presbyopes and may need enhancement if it persists beyond 6 months. Periodic cycloplegic refraction should be performed in these cases to check refractive stability.

Variable refraction can accompany development of haze and can be influenced by treatment with topical steroids. These cases can be difficult to manage when patients may be pushing for retreatment and feeling frustrated by fluctuating vision. Rarely, refractive instability may indicate corneal ectasia.

MANAGING EXPECTATIONS IN THE FIRST 6 MONTHS

The majority of patients will follow a usual postoperative course and may have minor concerns about dry eye or night vision recovery. However, a small percentage of patients will have more difficulty and concerns during the first few months after surface ablation (Table 8-3).

Patients will often be expecting discomfort and blurring in the first week but do not realize that it can take time for vision to sharpen.[3] Some patients will begin to panic if they are having visual disturbances after the first few weeks. A few patients will be inclined to record each refraction and to compare from visit to visit.

If there is a specific complication such as haze or significant dry eye, then additional time spent explaining these conditions may be needed. Technical staff can assist in educating the patients, but most patients would like to have face-to-face time with the surgeon if they feel they are not progressing as expected. Specific complications will be discussed in Chapter 10.

In many cases, there is no complication. Patients can have uncorrected acuities of 20/20 or better and complain of persistent ghosting or intermittent blur. It is rare for patients to require interim prescription eye wear; however, it can be helpful to discuss this as an option in appropriate cases.

TABLE 8-3. WHAT TO EXPECT IN THE FIRST 6 MONTHS FOLLOWING SURFACE ABLATION

- Vision: Worsening acuity for 1 to 4 days following surgery followed by gradual improvements over several weeks to months; expect fluctuations of vision, which will lessen over time. Night vision may take longer to improve. Enhancements can be considered after 6 months if the refraction is stable.

- Comfort: Comfort may worsen over the first 2 days and should improve by day 4 or 5 when contact is removed. Some foreign-body sensation may persist for days to weeks, especially in dry eye patients.

- Dry eye: Dry eye will improve over the first 3 to 6 months. Persistent dry eye is to be expected for patients with dry eye preoperatively and may need daily treatment on a permanent basis.

- Night vision: Night vision can take longer to improve and may be affected by residual refractive error. Most patients will notice improvement over the first month, although it may take longer for some patients.

- Reading vision: Even younger patients may complain of difficulty with close tasks and in particular with computer use in the first few weeks. Presbyopes and near presbyopes will have more difficulty and may need readers.

Most of these patients simply need reassurance that their vision is likely to improve either with natural healing over time or with a future enhancement. If enhancement is likely, then explaining to the patient the need for refractive stability and outlining a specific plan will help the patient cope with vision symptoms.

For example, the plan may be to check refraction every 6 weeks until stable for 2 or 3 consecutive visits, or if the patient is still on topical steroids, then the plan may be to wait up to 3 months following discontinuation of steroids to consider enhancement. Discussing the plan with the patient and documenting the plan in the chart will allow for a consistent message from visit to visit and will help the patient accept the need to wait for enhancement.

For persistently unhappy patients who have no obvious cause for vision disturbance, additional testing including a cycloplegic refraction should be done. Specialized testing, such as optical coherence tomography or visual fields, might also be useful in these cases (Figure 8-1).[4]

PATIENT SATISFACTION SURVEY

After 6 months, patients should be asked to complete an anonymous satisfaction survey (Figure 8-2). This allows patients to express any concerns they may have not been comfortable saying in person at an office visit. This also helps the surgeon and staff to recognize issues that may need to be corrected in the pre- and postoperative routines.

Most surgery centers are likely to have a high percentage of positive feedback but will have an opportunity to improve the quality of care by providing patients with the postoperative satisfaction survey. Some jurisdictions may require a patient survey for accreditation of the surgery center and may also require a specific protocol for patient complaints.

Patients should be encouraged to voice any concerns to the physician or office manager at any point in the process. Printed materials can also be used to provide patients with information about how to bring concerns to the attention of staff. Handling dissatisfaction or complaints successfully

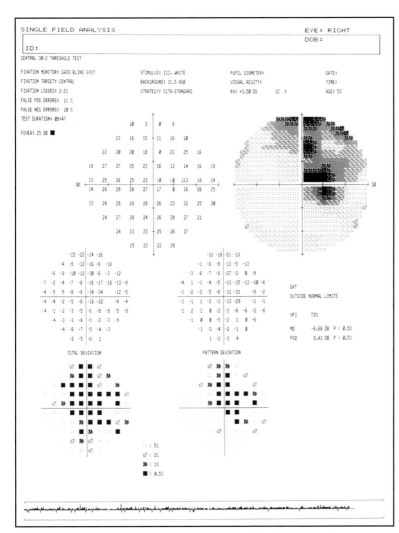

Figure 8-1. Special testing can be helpful in patients with persistent symptoms following surface ablation. This patient had persistent complaints of puffy lids and poor quality of vision following LASIK, describing the vision as "flat." There were no apparent abnormalities on examination and uncorrected acuities were 20/20 oculus uterque. On visual field testing, a significant disturbance was present and computed tomography revealed a large sphenoid wing meningioma with optic nerve compression.

can be a valuable asset to any practice as the unhappy patient who feels the staff has addressed concerns appropriately may refer future patients as a result.

SUMMARY

The majority of patients will have an uncomplicated postoperative course and a high level of satisfaction following surface ablation.[5] Providing patients with appropriate expectations and support when visual recovery is slower than anticipated will result in an overall higher level of satisfaction following surface ablation.

REFERENCES

1. Nien CJ, Flynn KJ, Chang M, Brown D, Jester JV. Reducing peak corneal haze after photorefractive keratectomy in rabbits: prednisolone acetate 1.00% versus cyclosporine A 0.05%. *J Cataract Refract Surg.* 2011;37(5):937-944.

PATIENT SATISFACTION SURVEY

This survey will be kept anonymous. Please answer honestly so we can improve our care and service to you. Specific comments will help us maintain and improve the quality of our care.

How would you rate the following, please circle your answer

Practice's overall performance:

Excellent   Fair   Poor

Ability to obtain an appointment in a time frame that met your expectation:

Excellent   Fair   Poor

Courteous and professional treatment by reception staff:

Excellent   Fair   Poor

Courteous and professional treatment by technical staff:

Excellent   Fair   Poor

Courteous and professional treatment by surgery staff:

Excellent   Fair   Poor

Courteous and professional treatment by the surgeon:

Excellent   Fair   Poor

Wait time to see the technician:

Excellent   Fair   Poor

Wait time to see the surgeon:

Excellent   Fair   Poor

Figure 8-2A. Sample patient satisfaction survey.

2. Murakami Y, Manche EE. Prospective, randomized comparison of self-reported postoperative dry eye and visual fluctuation in LASIK and photorefractive keratectomy. *Ophthalmology.* 2012;119(11):2220-2224.
3. Reilly CD, Panday V, Lazos V, Mittelstaedt BR. PRK vs LASEK vs Epi-LASIK: a comparison of corneal haze, postoperative pain and visual recovery in moderate to high myopia. *Nepal J Ophthalmol.* 2010;2(4):97-104.
4. Yamaguchi T, Murat D, Kimura I, et al. Diagnosis of steroid-induced glaucoma after photorefractive keratectomy. *J Refract Surg.* 2008;24(4):413-415.
5. Manche EE, Haw WW. Wavefront-guided laser in situ keratomileusis (Lasik) versus wavefront-guided photorefractive keratectomy (Prk): a prospective randomized eye-to-eye comparison (an American Ophthalmological Society thesis). *Trans Am Ophthalmol Soc.* 2011;109:201-220.

Thoroughly educated on my surgical procedure in a manner that I could understand.

Excellent   Fair   Poor

Thoroughly educated regarding my pre-operative instructions:

Excellent   Fair   Poor

Thoroughly educated regarding my post-operative instructions:

Excellent   Fair   Poor

My questions were answered to my satisfaction:

Excellent   Fair   Poor

Overall quality of care provided was:

Excellent   Fair   Poor

Additional Comments:
_____
_____
_____
_____
_____
_____
_____
_____
_____

How did you hear of Western Laser Eye Associates?

Referred   Website   Word of mouth   Other

Western Laser Eye Associates thank you for taking the time to complete our survey!

*Anonymous comments may be used on the web and/or other materials. If you wish to **not** have your comments posted please check the space provided _____*

Figure 8-2B. Sample patient satisfaction survey.

The Risk of Ectasia After Surface Ablation

Rupa D. Shah, MD and J. Bradley Randleman, MD

Postoperative ectasia (after corneal refractive surgery) is defined as progressive corneal steepening and warpage usually associated with increasing myopia and astigmatism, corneal thinning, and loss of uncorrected and spectacle-corrected acuity.[1] It is a rare but well-described complication of laser-assisted in situ keratomileusis (LASIK),[1-5] with identifiable preoperative risk factors in most cases, the most significant of which are 1) naturally occurring corneal ectatic disorders, including keratoconus and pellucid marginal corneal degeneration, 2) topographic abnormalities signifying early or abortive ectatic disease states such as forme fruste keratoconus, 3) young patient age, 4) thin corneas, and 5) insufficient residual stromal thickness.[6,7] Postoperative ectasia cases occurring after LASIK without apparent preoperative risk factors have also been reported.[7-10]

As compared with LASIK, the incidence appears much lower with only a handful of cases reported in the literature.[3,11-19] This difference could reflect under-reporting; however, because photorefractive keratectomy (PRK) was performed in greater abundance in the mid-1990s, before the advent of today's screening techniques, it is likely that if the incidence were higher, many more cases would have been reported from that time, which they were not. Therefore, it appears that there is a lower tendency for patients to develop ectasia after PRK.[20] Leccisotti[16] published an incidence of 0.03% from a retrospective, noncomparative case series of 6453 myopic eyes treated with PRK with a minimum follow-up of 18 months; however, all patients had keratoconus or forme fruste keratoconus preoperatively. In fact, the preponderance of postoperative ectasia after surface ablation have occurred in patients with abnormal preoperative topographies[3,11,13,14,16,17] or a positive family history of keratoconus.[15] Further, a variety of reports have demonstrated the development of ectasia after LASIK but not PRK in ipsilateral eyes of the same patients.[10,18] However, there are also reports of refractive and topographic stability after PRK in patients with abnormal topography or suspect keratoconus.[19,20]

Exacerbation of inherent biomechanical instability is the underlying mechanism for most cases of postoperative ectasia after laser vision correction. Keratoconic corneas are inherently weaker than normal corneas[21] and, after laser vision correction, the ablation of the anterior stroma can compound any inherent biomechanical weakness.[22] The anterior one-third of the cornea has the greatest biomechanical strength[23]; thus, even with surface ablation techniques and minimal refractive error correction, Bowman's and the strongest, most anterior stromal fibers are ablated. Therefore, screening for inherent biomechanical weakness remains of the utmost importance even for surface ablation cases.

Controversy exists regarding the risk of developing ectasia after surface ablation techniques, including photorefractive keratectomy (PRK). Some surgeons consider performing PRK in eyes in which they might not perform LASIK.[7,20,24] Indeed, many of the risk factors for LASIK, including the interrelationship between high myopia, thin corneas, and low residual stromal bed thickness, should be minimized with surface ablation. However, patients with significant topographic abnormalities are likely still at an increased risk for postoperative ectasia and in these patients, surgery should only be undertaken in special circumstances and with unique informed consent.

A large part of the controversy surrounding the safety of surface ablation in corneas with abnormal topographies is our still-growing understanding of corneal biomechanics and the evaluation of what is really an abnormally weak cornea as opposed to one with topographic changes in the absence of true weakening. As technology advances, it may become easier to accurately delineate these groups and thereby offer surgery to more patients who appear abnormal using our current screening algorithms but likely do not suffer any reduction in actual biomechanical integrity.

Summary

Corneal ectasia can occur after PRK, especially in individuals with abnormal topography, although the occurrence appears significantly lower than after LASIK. Patients should be screened using the same methodology for topographic image review as for LASIK as the same risk factors exist for surface ablation. Refractive surgeons should be aware of the potential of development of ectasia even after surface ablation and should counsel their patients accordingly.

REFERENCES

1. Randleman JB, Russell B, Ward MA, Thompson KP, Stulting RD. Risk factors and prognosis for corneal ectasia after LASIK. *Ophthalmology.* 2003;110(2):267-275.

2. Argento C, Cosentino MJ, Tytiun A, Rapetti G, Zarate J. Corneal ectasia after laser in situ keratomileusis. *J Cataract Refract Surg.* 2001;27(9):1440-1448.

3. Holland SP, Srivannaboon S, Reinstein DZ. Avoiding serious corneal complications of laser assisted in situ keratomileusis and photorefractive keratectomy. *Ophthalmology.* 2000;107(4):640-652.

4. Pallikaris IG, Kymionis GD, Astyrakakis NI. Corneal ectasia induced by laser in situ keratomileusis. *J Cataract Refract Surg.* 2001;27(11):1796-1802.

5. Seiler T, Quurke AW. Iatrogenic keratectasia after LASIK in a case of forme fruste keratoconus. *J Cataract Refract Surg.* 1998;24(7):1007-1009.

6. Randleman JB, Trattler WB, Stulting RD. Validation of the Ectasia Risk Score System for preoperative laser in situ keratomileusis screening. *Am J Ophthalmol.* 2008;145(5):813-818.

7. Randleman JB, Woodward M, Lynn MJ, Stulting RD. Risk assessment for ectasia after corneal refractive surgery. *Ophthalmology.* 2008;115(1):37-50.

8. Ambrosio R Jr, Dawson DG, Salomao M, et al. Corneal ectasia after LASIK despite low preoperative risk: tomographic and biomechanical findings in the unoperated, stable, fellow eye. *J Refract Surg.* 2010;26(11):906-911.

9. Amoils SP, Deist MB, Gous P, Amoils PM. Iatrogenic keratectasia after laser in situ keratomileusis for less than -4.0 to -7.0 diopters of myopia. *J Cataract Refract Surg.* 2000;26(7):967-977.

10. Hodge C, Lawless M, Sutton G. Keratectasia following LASIK in a patient with uncomplicated PRK in the fellow eye. *J Cataract Refract Surg.* 2011;37(3):603-607.

11. Lovisolo CF, Fleming JF. Intracorneal ring segments for iatrogenic keratectasia after laser in situ keratomileusis or photorefractive keratectomy. *J Refract Surg.* 2002;18(5):535-541.

12. Parmar D, Claoué C. Keratectasia following excimer laser photorefractive keratectomy. *Acta Ophthalmol Scand.* 2004;82(1):102-105.

13. Malecaze F, Coullet J, Calvas P, Fournié P, Arné JL, Brodaty C. Corneal ectasia after photorefractive keratectomy for low myopia. *Ophthalmology.* 2006;113(5):742-746.

14. Reznik J, Salz JJ, Klimava A. Development of unilateral corneal ectasia after PRK with ipsilateral preoperative forme fruste keratoconus. *J Refract Surg.* 2008;24(8):843-847.

15. Navas A, Ariza E, Haber A, Fermón S, Velázquez R, Suárez R. Bilateral keratectasia after photorefractive keratectomy. *J Refract Surg.* 2007;23(9):941-943.

16. Leccisotti A. Corneal ectasia after photorefractive keratectomy. *Graefes Arch Clin Exp Ophthalmol.* 2007;245(6):869-875.

17. Randleman JB, Caster AI, Banning CS, Stulting RD. Corneal ectasia after photorefractive keratectomy. *J Cataract Refract Surg.* 2006;32(8):1395-1398.

18. Kymionis GD, Tsiklis N, Karp CL, Kalyvianaki M, Pallikaris AI. Unilateral corneal ectasia after laser in situ keratomileusis in a patient with uncomplicated photorefractive keratectomy in the fellow eye. *J Cataract Refract Surg.* 2007;33(5):859-861.

19. Spadea L. Collagen crosslinking for ectasia following PRK performed in excimer laser-assisted keratoplasty for keratoconus. *Eur J Ophthalmology.* 2011;22(2):274-277.

20. Hardten DR, Gosavi VV. Photorefractive keratectomy in eyes with atypical topography. *J Cataract Refract Surg.* 2009;35(8):1437-1444.

21. Andreassen TT, Simonsen AH, Oxlund H. Biomechanical properties of keratoconus and normal corneas. *Exp Eye Res.* 1980;31(4):435-441.

22. Dupps WJ Jr, Roberts C. Effect of acute biomechanical changes on corneal curvature after photokeratectomy. *J Refract Surg.* 2001;17(6):658-669.

23. Randleman JB, Dawson DG, Grossniklaus HE, McCarey BE, Edelhauser HF. Depth-dependent cohesive tensile strength in human donor corneas: implications for refractive surgery. *J Refract Surg.* 2008;24(1):S85-S89.

24. Binder PS, Lindstrom RL, Stulting RD, et al. Keratoconus and corneal ectasia after LASIK. *J Cataract Refract Surg.* 2005;31(11):2035-2038.

9

Retreatment Following Surface Ablation

One of the factors in predicting satisfaction is enhancement. When or whether to do enhancement has to be considered on a case-by-case basis. It is helpful to set expectations for surgery prior to the primary treatment to avoid dissatisfaction due to unrealistic goals on the part of the patient. For example, uncorrected acuity will not be better than best-corrected visual acuity (BCVA) in most cases.

Enhancement policies will also vary between surgeons or surgery centers. Patients need to know if enhancements are covered in the initial fee and, if so, for what period of time postoperatively. Some centers have a base price for the primary surgery and offer "insurance" on top of that initial fee to cover enhancements or the patient is charged a larger fee for enhancement if he or she does not have the "insurance" up front. Due to this variability, it is important to clarify these policies in advance of the initial treatment.

ENHANCEMENT CRITERIA

Setting appropriate expectations before primary surface ablation will make the decision about whether or not to enhance easier (Table 9-1). Reinforcing that the goal of surgery is to provide vision similar to what the patient had prior to surgery with glasses or contact lenses and taking care not to overpromise will help to avoid inappropriate expectations.

Some surgeons will have a specific cut-off of when they might consider enhancement, such as 0.75 D of residual myopia or a vision level such as 20/20 (Figure 9-1).[1,2] It is important to consider the specifics of each case and to check the cycloplegic refraction prior to deciding if enhancement should be performed.

In general, it may not be wise to consider enhancement for uncorrected acuity of 20/20, as a small residual enhancement may not necessarily improve binocular function and could, in rare cases, reduce the uncorrected distance vision result. For example, treatment for residual hyperopia may leave a patient slightly myopic as a result or correcting a very small amount of residual myopia in a presbyope may impact the uncorrected distance vision.

Reminding the patient not to compare eyes by covering or closing one eye repeatedly is often necessary. The goal is to provide good binocular vision and not necessarily for the 2 eyes to be

Anderson Penno EE. *Surface Ablation:*
Techniques for Optimum Results (pp 109-115).
© 2013 SLACK Incorporated.

TABLE 9-1. SAMPLE ENHANCEMENT CRITERIA

- Uncorrected visual acuity (UCVA) <20/20
- Residual refraction >0.75 D
- Refractive stability on 2 visits >1 month apart
- At least 6 months postoperative
- Binocular acuity affected (not just noticing when one eye covered)
- Satisfactory ocular surface free of tear film abnormalities

Figure 9-1. This patient had UCVA 20/20[-1] but consistently complained about distance acuity ocular sinister (OS). Enhancement of this mild mixed astigmatism led to UCVA of 20/15 and satisfaction with the final outcome.

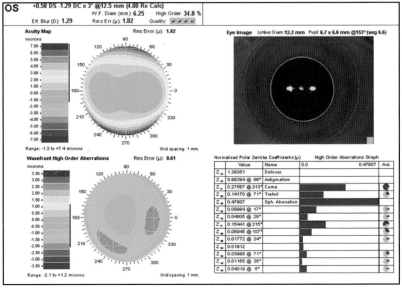

subjectively exactly the same. Repeatedly checking will cause the patient to be more aware of differences and working with both eyes together will allow the patient to adjust to small differences between eyes.

If the uncorrected acuity is the same or better than the preoperative BCVA and if the patient is not symptomatic with both eyes working together, then enhancement may not be necessary. It may be useful to also repeat a cycloplegic refraction to verify there is no unexpected hyperopia. Most people are very reasonable regarding advice for or against enhancement.

Occasionally, a patient has unrealistic expectations about timing or need for enhancement. It is important to not rush into enhancement too early or if there are other issues, such as dry eye, regression, or corneal haze, that need attention first. Extra time may be needed to be sure the patient fully understands recommendations for or against enhancement. For small enhancements, it is important to caution the patient that the vision may be worse than before enhancement for days to weeks.

Marketing can play a role in expectations. Advertisements that give a "20/20" guarantee or promise vision that is better than what can be achieved with glasses or contacts may lead the patient to have unrealistic goals for surgery. Even if these ads are not from your practice, if these types of ads are common in your community, you may need to address these prior to primary surgery. While most patients will achieve 20/20 or better uncorrected acuity and some will find their vision improved from prior best-corrected, it is not possible to guarantee these results.

ENHANCEMENTS AND AGE

In presbyopic or near-presbyopic patients with residual myopia, an enhancement may improve distance vision at the expense of close vision.[3] Even when monovision was not the intended target, some of these patients will be satisfied to retain a small amount of myopia in one or both eyes. Enhancements following presbyopia-correcting intraocular lenses can be effective in improving visual function and patient satisfaction.[4] This will depend entirely on patient age, occupation, and hobbies.

For a patient who is doing well for all activities with the exception of night driving, a pair of glasses for that activity might be preferable to an enhancement, which would require reading glasses for close work. Showing the correction in a trial frame or even a contact lens trial might be helpful in these cases.

For intentional monovision cases where the patient is complaining about distance vision, the distance eye should be enhanced if needed prior to correcting the reading eye for distance. Many centers will have an extra charge in this case if one eye was intentionally under-corrected for monovision and the patient later changes his or her mind. In most cases, a contact lens trial or showing the correction in a trial frame will avoid this situation.

It is typical to have some hyperopia in the first weeks following surface ablation. Patients of all ages will often complain about computer work in particular. For young patients, there may be an intentional target for mild hyperopia due to the fact that natural progression in myopes may tend to cause them to drift more myopic over time. Most younger patients will tolerate mild residual hyperopia without any problems.

Near or early presbyopes can be more difficult. In spite of symptoms, the patient should be counseled to wait until the refraction is stable. For mild residual hyperopia that persists, enhancement should be done if it will improve distance acuity. Dependence on reading glasses is expected. Presbyopes who work full correction for distance prior to surgery will usually have appropriate expectations, but spectacle wearers will sometimes have more difficulty adjusting. This is particularly true for mild myopia preoperatively.

EYE DOMINANCE

Eye dominance should be considered in any decision for enhancement. If uncorrected distance acuity is reduced compared to preoperative best-corrected acuity in the dominant eye, then a small enhancement is more likely to be of benefit. If the nondominant eye has only a small residual correction, then it may not be necessary to enhance. In general, if the patient is happy with his or her vision working with both eyes together, then enhancement may not be necessary.

As a general rule, many ophthalmologists and optometrists will recommend the dominant eye be corrected for distance if monovision is targeted. However, a contact lens trial either way prior to surgery is recommended if possible as some people will prefer the dominant eye for near.

DRY EYE

Dry eye can be a confounding condition in patients with mild residual correction following surface ablation. It is a common reason for patients to be unhappy with their vision even if they have excellent Snellen acuity and plano or near-plano refractions.[5] Treatment of dry eye prior to considering enhancement will improve the ultimate outcome even if this may result in a delay of enhancement.

Fluctuating vision may be present due to unstable tear film. Patients may not recognize this can be a symptom of dry eye and may think that this indicates a need for enhancement. Treatment of coexisting allergies or blepharitis is often required. Educating the patient will help with compliance in treatment and will help him or her understand why enhancement may not be recommended or why it may be delayed.

While topical cyclosporine A has not necessarily been demonstrated to be of benefit for prophylactic use, it may be helpful for postoperative patients who are struggling with dry eye. In these cases, consideration of enhancement should be delayed in order to allow for the use of cyclosporine A drops for 3 to 6 months as it can take some time for the benefit of this medication to become apparent. Similarly, punctal plugs or oral supplementation with flax oil and fish oil can be tried in advance of consideration of enhancement.

In many cases, patients will have a history of dry eye or other ocular surface disease prior to surface ablation. They may need to be reminded that dry eye is a chronic condition that can require daily treatment.

ENHANCEMENT TIMING

Many surgeons wait a minimum of 6 months before performing enhancement. By notifying the patient prior to surgery that you will not consider enhancement for up to 6 months, the patient will have the proper expectations and understand the need to be patient with the healing process. This allows for complete corneal nerve recovery and epithelial remodeling. In addition, treatment for ocular surface disease can be implemented if necessary during the postoperative period.

A tapering dose of topical steroid is often recommended following uncomplicated surface ablation, which may last for 4 months, and a 6-month time frame allows for stability to be verified following discontinuation of the steroid. This is outlined in Chapter 8.

There are reasons why enhancement may have to be delayed (Table 9-2). Patients with haze may have to wait a considerable length of time prior to considering enhancement. Haze prevention and treatment will be discussed in Chapter 10. Enhancement may also have to be delayed for treatment of dry eye. Hyperopia following a high myopic treatment may also warrant a longer period of time prior to considering enhancement. Cycloplegic refraction is necessary in order to confirm stability.

Enhancement policies will differ between surgeons and centers. Some centers will include enhancement for a specific length of time, such as 18 months. Patients should be clear on these policies before the primary surgery. Some patients with mild residual refractive error may have a hard time deciding if they wish to enhance or not. Having a time frame in place can be helpful in encouraging a decision and avoids the need to do repeated exams over several months while the patient tries to make a choice.

REFRACTIVE STABILITY

Immediately following surface ablation, some hyperopia may be expected with a mild myopic shift over the first months. For most uncomplicated cases, the refraction will stabilize by 6 months and should be verified by serial refractions with at least one cycloplegic refraction prior to considering enhancement. This is important in young patients who may easily measure more minus on refraction due to robust accommodative amplitudes and also for older patients to deduce latent hyperopia. For uncomplicated cases, enhancements can be done within the first 18 months following primary surface ablation.

There have been centers that offer a lifetime enhancement. A few patients will return many years later asking for enhancement. For surface ablation, enhancement can be done many years

TABLE 9-2. CONSIDERATIONS FOR DELAY OF ENHANCEMENT

- Corneal haze: Corneal haze may need prolonged treatment with topical steroids and may influence refraction; enhancement should be delayed pending stabilization of refraction and discontinuation of topical steroids.

- Significant dry eye: Dry eye can reduce BCVA and can create refractive and topographic instability; improvement of ocular surface prior to enhancement will improve ultimate success.

- Regression: Highly myopic corrections may regress beyond 6 months.

- Mild myopia: For presbyopes or near presbyopes, mild myopia may be an asset to near vision; patients who are not under pressure to decide about enhancement within a specific time frame may ultimately decide not to undergo enhancement.

TABLE 9-3. CAUSES FOR REFRACTIVE INSTABILITY FOLLOWING SURFACE ABLATION

- One to 6 months postoperatively: Normal initial hyperopic shift followed by mild myopic shift, fluctuations due to dry eye, regression, haze, ectasia

- Six to 12 months postoperatively: Continued regression following high myopic correction, haze, ectasia

- Instability following initial stability: Sudden shifts can indicate diabetes; slower progression may be measured in cataracts or latent hyperopia, ectasia

later without increasing the risk of retreatment. However, there can be some concerns with patients who present years later for enhancement. In most cases, there will have been a shift in the refraction, which has prompted the patient to desire enhancement.

If the refraction is not stable, there may be early cataract development. Diabetes should also be ruled out for patients with significant or sudden shifts (Table 9-3). If possible, documentation of refractions for the past few years can be helpful in determining refractive stability. If there is a very slow progression of myopia, an enhancement could be considered; however, the patient should understand that repeated enhancements are not recommended. If there is rapid progression, enhancement may not be recommended and alternatives such as cataract surgery may be necessary. In rare cases, ectasia should be considered.

ENHANCEMENT TECHNIQUE

Surface ablation has the advantage of the simplicity of retreatment. Although laser-assisted in situ keratomileusis (LASIK) flaps can be lifted in many cases even years after surgery, there can be difficulties with flaps that are too adherent to lift and with epithelial ingrowth following LASIK enhancement. For surface ablation, the retreatment involves epithelial removal in the same manner as described in Chapter 4 with the exception that the epikeratome cannot be used for retreatments.

Epithelial laser in situ keratomileusis (epi-LASIK) enhancements must be done with a brush or alcohol-assisted technique because the microkeratome relies on an intact Bowman's layer in order

Figure 9-2. Epi-LASIK enhancements must be done with a brush or alcohol-assisted technique because the microkeratome relies on an intact Bowman's layer in order to function correctly. (Photograph by Amanda Sneddon.)

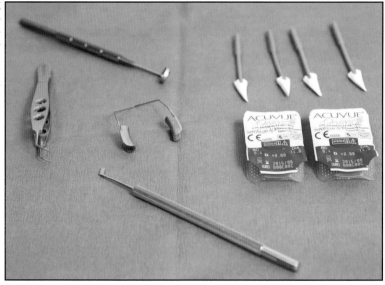

TABLE 9-4. CONSIDERATIONS FOR ENHANCEMENT FOLLOWING SURFACE ABLATION

• Expectations	• Age
• Timing of enhancement	• Eye dominance
• Refractive stability	• Dry eye

to function correctly (Figure 9-2). For single eye enhancements, a longer recovery of best vision compared to the primary epi-LASIK is usually not troubling to the patient as he or she is functional with the fellow eye.

Retreatment considerations include timing, refractive stability, patient age, eye dominance, dry eye, and patient satisfaction (Table 9-4).

UNILATERAL VERSUS BILATERAL ENHANCEMENT

In many cases, only one eye may be in need of enhancement, but there are some cases where residual correction may be present bilaterally. Often, it is reasonable to consider enhancement in one eye at a time due to factors such as mild residual myopia in a presbyope or in cases of residual hyperopia that is more prominent in one eye. In these cases, enhancement in one eye may be all that is needed to provide good binocular function.

In cases of unexpected over- or undercorrection, regression, or haze, it is prudent to enhance one eye at a time in order to preserve functioning during the healing period for the enhanced eye. If only one eye is recommended for enhancement due to unexpected results, then the second eye should be delayed until the stability and results of the first enhancement are verified. Most patients will find their functioning is better during the recovery period when only one eye is treated.

Although patients will be legal to drive in the majority of cases due to the vision in the untreated eye, they should be encouraged to limit driving until the contact lens is removed from the enhanced eye. Contact lens shift or photophobia may impact binocular function, which may affect activities such as driving or computer use. Patients will still have to factor recovery of the enhanced eye into their return to work, although in general, patients are often back to usual activities sooner after a unilateral surface ablation procedure.

SUMMARY

Uncorrected residual refractive error is the most common cause for dissatisfaction following refractive surgery. Communicating enhancement policies preoperatively will assist in postoperative management.

REFERENCES

1. Sharma N, Balasubramanya R, Sinha R, Titiyal JS, Vajpayee RB. Retreatment of LASIK. *J Refractive Surg.* 2006;22(4):396-401.
2. Gabler B, Winkler von Mohrenfels C, Herrmann W, Gora F, Lohmann CP. Laser-assisted subepithelial keratectomy enhancement of residual myopia after primary myopic LASEK: six-month results in 10 eyes. *J Cataract Refract Surg.* 2003;29(7):1260-1266.
3. Garcia-Gonzalez M, Teus MA, Hernandez-Verdejo JL. Visual outcomes of LASIK-induced monovision in myopic patients with presbyopia. *Am J Ophthalmol.* 2010;150(3):381-386.
4. Macsai MS, Fontes BM. Refractive enhancement following presbyopia-correcting intraocular lens implantation. *Curr Opin Ophthalmol.* 2008;19(1):18-21.
5. Shtein RM. Post-LASIK dry eye. *Expert Rev Ophthalmol.* 2011;6(5):575-582.

Complications of Surface Ablation

The rate of complications following surface ablation is low but it is not zero. Many patients choose surface ablation specifically for the low complication rate.[1] Others may be recommended to have surface ablation due to thin corneas. Most complications of surface ablation can be avoided with careful preoperative selection or can be treated to avoid loss of best-corrected acuity.

EARLY POSTOPERATIVE COMPLICATIONS

Pain and Photophobia

Pain, vision fluctuations, photophobia, and foreign-body sensation are expected and should not be considered complications (Table 10-1). There is a wide range of experiences within the normal range. Some patients have only minor discomfort in the range of what it feels like to sleep in contacts. Others may have enough pain that they have to stay in a dark room.

Frequent gentle ice packs, frequent preservative-free tears, and oral pain medication will be sufficient in combination with advice to rest and spend time with the eyes closed. For most patients, discomfort will increase after 24 hours postoperatively. Discomfort will usually worsen during the second 24 hours before improving in a typical case.

In addition to oral pain medication, some patients can benefit from a mild sedative, such as 1 mg lorazepam at bedtime or a sleep aid.

Adverse Drug Reactions

Oral Medication

Oral pain medications may result in nausea and vomiting in some patients. Patients should be cautioned about possible side effects of all medications and should be instructed to discontinue the medication and call if a reaction occurs. Instruct the patient about possible interactions with over-the-counter medications and review any prescription medications being used.

Benzodiazepam sedatives are generally well tolerated in the low doses usually used on the day of surgery. A few patients will experience some imbalance as a result of taking a benzodiazepam

Anderson Penno EE. *Surface Ablation:*
Techniques for Optimum Results (pp 117-126).
© 2013 SLACK Incorporated.

TABLE 10-1. EARLY POSTOPERATIVE COMPLICATIONS

• Excessive pain and photophobia	• Delayed re-epithelialization
• Adverse drug reaction	• Epithelial shift/loose epithelium
• Noninfectious keratitis	• Corneal edema
• Infectious keratitis	• Large fusion pattern

and in rare cases can experience significant dizziness. Patients should avoid alcohol after taking a sedative. Patients should be cautioned about possible adverse side effects of oral medication and should be accompanied by a companion on the day of surgery.

Topical Medication

There have been sporadic reports of corneal infiltrates, corneal thinning, and corneal melt associated with topical nonsteroidal anti-inflammatory drops.[2] This is uncommon but topical medications should be considered in any case of early postoperative keratitis.[3]

Tetracaine minums are often given to postoperative patients to use sparingly in the first 48 hours. Overuse of a topical anesthetic may be associated with delayed epithelial healing and could mask symptoms of infection. To avoid overuse, patients are cautioned and typically only 1 or 2 minums are dispensed to the patient.

Infectious Keratitis

A recent retrospective analysis of more than 18,000 eyes reported a 0.2% rate of infectious keratitis following surface ablation (Table 10-2).[4] The most common organism isolated was *Staphylococcus aureus*, although more than half of the cases were culture negative. Prevention of infectious keratitis will include appropriate surgical techniques and covering the patient with a topical antibiotic while the epithelial defect is healing.

Many surgeons use a fourth-generation fluoroquinolone for coverage during re-epithelialization. While these are broad-spectrum antibiotics with good gram-positive coverage and coverage for some atypical organisms, there has been reported resistance in *aureus* and *Pseudomonas aeruginosa*. It is imperative to follow postoperative surface ablation cases closely in the first few days to detect infection early.

Because the usual signs and symptoms of corneal infection may be masked by the typical pain and blurred vision to be expected in the first few days following surgery, a slit-lamp examination at 24 to 48 hours after treatment is a good practice. This will allow for detection of corneal infiltrates early and for changes in drops to provide additional coverage. Patients should also be counseled to report any significant discharge that develops.

Adding a combination antibiotic treatment or fortified antibiotic, discontinuing nonsteroidal anti-inflammatory drops, and altering the frequency of topical steroids may be necessary. Daily slit-lamp examination may be needed, and cultures should be performed in cases that are not responding quickly to topical treatment.

Noninfectious Keratitis

Noninfectious infiltrates will usually be peripheral and less dense than infectious infiltrates, although all infiltrates should be considered potentially infectious with frequent examinations until clearing. Discontinuing nonsteroidal anti-inflammatory drops, increasing topical steroids, and switching to preservative-free drops may be needed.

TABLE 10-2. INFECTIOUS KERATITIS

• *Staphylococcus aureus* (most common isolate) • Culture-negative (>50%)	• *Pseudomonas aeruginosa* • Atypical organisms

Tight contact lenses may contribute to infiltrates. Removal or removal and replacement of bandage contact lenses may be needed but can result in shifting of the underlying epithelium if a defect is still present. For smaller defects, removal of the bandage contact lens with a pressure patch application overnight can be effective.

Loose Epithelium/Epithelial Shift

If the bandage contact lens shifts or if the contact falls out and has to be replaced, the epithelium may shift within the treatment zone. There may be a history of accidently rubbing the eye, or it may occur spontaneously. Most often, the patient will report a sudden significant increase in pain, photophobia, tearing, and worsening vision.

If the shifted area is small and the contact lens is still in position, then leaving the bandage lens in place should be considered. Complete re-epithelialization will likely be delayed, and the resulting fusion line may be larger, which will slow recovery of best acuity. However, in most cases, when the contact is removed, a larger area of epithelium will shift.

For larger areas of epithelial shifting or if the contact is out of position or has fallen out, the remaining epithelium may need to be débrided and repositioned at the slit-lamp or at the operating microscope. Fragments of epithelium should be removed, and folded epithelial edges should be smoothed. If at all possible, any loose sheets of epithelium that are simply shifted but are not torn should be smoothed rather than removed. When attempting to remove a loose epithelium with a forceps, the defect will often extend or tear. A smaller edge fold can be left if it is outside the visual axis.

If there are fragments of epithelium in the defect zone, the new epithelium will grow over them, leaving an irregular surface. If there is a small fragment outside the visual axis that ends up under the new epithelium, it can be left in place and it will smooth out over several weeks. Any fragments left centrally should be débrided.

To avoid reabrasion after the contact lens is removed, a complete fusion line should be present before removing the contact. It is tempting to remove the contact when there is only a tiny defect present, but this can result in re-abrasion shortly thereafter. Leaving the contact in another day will avoid a setback of a larger area of loose epithelium.

Patients should be advised not to rub the eyes and use frequent artificial tears for the remainder of the day following contact removal. If there is an elevated fusion line or irregular epithelium centrally, then ointment should be instilled just after contact removal in order to avoid reabrasion. Reabrasion will need to be treated as described above with débridement and contact lens replacement.

Delayed Re-Epithelialization

Slow resolution of the epithelial defect can be frustrating for the patient and the surgeon but does not necessarily affect the final visual outcome. As described above, shifted epithelium or reabrasion can result in delayed re-epithelialization (Table 10-3). In some cases, healing is simply slower than usual with no apparent cause.

TABLE 10-3. CAUSES FOR DELAYED RE-EPITHELIALIZATION

• Shifted epithelium	• Overuse of topical anesthetic
• Reabrasion	• Preservative sensitivity

Reducing the frequency of topical steroids and using preservative-free drops should be considered. Overuse of topical anesthetic may be a factor and should be discontinued if the patient is using these drops. Higher corrections with mitomycin C use may be expected to re-epithelialize more slowly.

As long as there are no infiltrates and the epithelium is advancing even slowly, then the contact should be left in place with slit-lamp examination every 1 or 2 days. Removing the contact lens and placing a pressure patch may be necessary in rare cases. The pressure patch should be replaced with a corneal exam daily.

Corneal Edema

Corneal edema may be present in the first 48 hours and will typically resolve when the epithelial defect is healed. This is more likely to be present with higher corrections but less commonly is seen even with low corrections. There is usually no need to change medications if the epithelium is healing as expected. Addition of muro-128 drops or ointment can be considered if corneal edema persists after the contact lens is removed, which would be rare. Corneal edema can cause the visual acuity to be very poor (20/200 or worse), and these patients may need reassurance that the vision will recover.

Persistent Fusion Line

The differences in acuity and in quality of vision between epi-LASIK and other methods of epithelial removal within the first several days to weeks are due to the size of the fusion line. In general, epi-LASIK will result in a smaller linear fusion line as compared to a larger stellate fusion pattern with other methods of epithelial removal. The larger and more centrally located the fusion line is, the more visual disturbance will be present.

In general, the visual quality will improve over the first few days to few weeks after contact lens removal as the fusion line smooths out due to epithelial remodeling. If the fusion line is very large or in some cases just due to variation in healing, the fusion line is visible for weeks after surgery. This will result in complaints of blurred vision, ghosting, and in some cases measureable astigmatism even if no astigmatism was present preoperatively.

Switching to a nonpreserved steroid and continuing nonpreserved artificial tears may help speed recovery. Persistent fusion lines will generally resolve over several weeks and concurrently the patient symptoms improve and astigmatism resolves. These cases may require additional examinations to reassure the patient. Supporting the patient with additional documentation for delayed return to work or modified duties can help reduce patient stress. Treatment of dry eye will also be beneficial.

Persistent fusion lines are more likely to be seen in patients who have had an epithelial shift or reabrasion. They can be present even after uncomplicated surface ablation. Fortunately, persistent fusion line is more often unilateral and can explain differences in early postoperative acuity. In rare cases, it may take up to 6 months for visual symptoms to resolve.

TABLE 10-4. LATE POSTOPERATIVE COMPLICATIONS	
• Persistent dry eye	• Haze
• Night vision disturbances	• Recurrent erosion

LATE POSTOPERATIVE COMPLICATIONS

A small percentage of eyes will need enhancement for over- or undercorrection following surface ablation. This is not a complication and is expected due to differences in healing and response to the laser.

Dry Eye

Dry eye is the most common side effect of any type of laser vision correction (Table 10-4). Often, patients with significant dry eye postoperatively had dry eye prior to surgery. For full-time eyeglass wearers, the eyes may be drier due to the fact they no longer have the protective effects of wearing glasses. Glasses prevent evaporation and protect the eyes from wind and airborne particles. Contact lens wearers may also notice more sensitivity due to the exposure of the corneal surface following surface ablation.

Forewarning patients will allow them to be prepared for this possible side effect from surgery. Patients who are wishing to have surface ablation due to dry eye with contacts should be advised that surface ablation will not prevent dry eye. Mild dry eye can be treated with artificial tears as needed (Table 10-5).

Common sense measures, such as wearing sunglasses when lighting is appropriate, avoiding the use of dash heat or air conditioning in the car, and taking breaks from prolonged reading or computer work, may be helpful. Blink rate is measurably lower when concentrating on visually demanding tasks. Here is an easy-to-remember reminder: 20-20-20—every 20 minutes look away 20 feet and blink 20 times. This reminder will help to relax ciliary muscles and blinking helps relieve dry eye.

More significant dry eye will need daily treatment with artificial tears and treatment of coexisting conditions, such as meibomian dysfunction, should be addressed. Most importantly, dry eye and associated ocular surface dysfunction will require a change in daily routine. Using warm compresses for 3 to 5 minutes twice per day with artificial tears 2 to 4 times per day is a usual starting recommendation.

It is essential for patients to understand the need to develop a habit of treatment and that each intervention may take up to 6 or 8 weeks to provide maximum benefit. In order to maintain the benefit, treatment needs to be ongoing.

Moving to a gel lubricant at bedtime may be needed for some patients. Oral supplementation with a combination of flaxseed oil and fish oil may help improve tear quality. Some patients may need to stay with preservative-free artificial tears if they find they need them very frequently throughout the day.

Tear quantity may be improved with punctal plugs. Temporary dissolvable plugs may be helpful in the first few months if there is a possibility that dry eye may improve with corneal nerve recovery in the first few months following surface ablation. Temporary plugs will also help determine if side effects, such as tearing, are present before moving to a permanent punctal plug.

Topical cyclosporine A may be needed in more significant dry eye situations, although it is important for the patient to understand that this topical medication may make symptoms worse before they get better. It may also be necessary to use this medication for 3 to 6 months to obtain maximum benefit and the medication will need to be continued to maintain the effects.

TABLE 10-5. TREATMENT OF DRY EYE	
Mild	Regular use of artificial tears
	Treatment of coexisting conditions such as allergies
	Treatment of meibomian dysfunction with warm compresses
Moderate	Continue artificial tears and compresses and increase frequency
	Add gel at bedtime
	Add oral flax/fish oil supplements
	Encourage more breaks from prolonged close work
	Humidify environment
	Encourage sunglasses where appropriate
	Add topical cyclosporine
Severe	Switch to preservative-free tears with increased frequency
	Consider punctal plugs
	Consider plano spectacles to help prevent evaporation
	Consider night moisture goggles
	Prevent severe dry eye postoperatively by disqualifying patients with significant dry eye preoperatively

Educating patients about the complexity of the tear film and about the role of the lids and disorders affecting the meibomian glands in dry eye and discussing tear quantity versus tear quality will help to improve compliance with treatment recommendations.

The best way to prevent significant dry eye following surface ablation is to treat dry eye preoperatively and to avoid surgery in patients with significant untreated dry eye preoperatively. In particular, contact lens-intolerant patients should be approached with caution.

Recurrent Erosion

Persistent recurrent erosion is an uncommon complication of surface ablation. Pre-existing basement membrane dystrophy or postoperative corneal ulcer may be predisposing factors. Treatment includes topical lubrication and muro-128 ointment at bedtime. In most cases, daily use can prevent recurrences.

For persistent recurrent erosion, retreatment options may include PTK as discussed in Chapter 5.

Haze

Haze remains an uncommon but serious complication of surface ablation. Modification of treatment zones and ablation patterns since the introduction of PRK over 25 years ago has lessened haze frequency to a small percentage of postoperative patients.

Corneal haze following surface ablation involves a complex inflammatory cascade provoked by epithelial damage and apoptosis in combination with basement membrane and stromal injury. Fibroblasts migrate to the central cornea and transform into myofibroblasts, which results in irregularity and opacity.

Depending on the excimer laser platform in use, surgeons may routinely use mitomycin C intraoperatively as discussed in Chapter 6 for haze prevention. A tapering dose of topical steroid is often recommended for 4 to 6 months following surface ablation to prevent significant haze.

TABLE 10-6. CORNEAL HAZE GRADING	
STAGE	**SLIT-LAMP APPEARANCE**
0	Clear cornea
0.5	Trace haze seen with oblique illumination
1	Haze not interfering with iris detail visibility
2	Haze with mild obscuration of iris detail visibility
3	Haze with moderate obscuration of iris detail visibility
4	Complete opacity of the stroma

Adapted from Fantes FE, Hanna KD, Waring GO III, Pouliquen Y, Thompson KP, Savoldelli M. Wound healing after excimer laser keratomileusis (photorefractive keratectomy) in monkeys. *Arch Ophthalmol.* 1990;108(5):665-675.

Shifted epithelium and delayed re-epithelialization may increase risk of haze. Higher treatments and smaller optical zones have been associated with increased risk of haze. There are reports that hormonal changes and ultraviolet light may be inciting factors.

Fantes and colleagues published a haze grading scale that helps the clinician quantify haze at the slit-lamp (Table 10-6).[5] Optical coherence tomography can also be used to image haze.

Transitory Haze

Visually insignificant haze is common and will generally develop within a few months after surgery and will resolve over several months. Topical corticosteroids may have some beneficial effects in the treatment of visually significant haze; however, patients on topical steroids should be carefully monitored for increased intraocular pressure. Use of vitamin C has not been shown conclusively to reduce haze formation.

Late Haze

In contrast to transitory haze, late haze will develop after 2 to 5 months and is more likely to be visually significant.[6] Late haze may respond to topical steroids but may persist for up to 3 years (Figure 10-1). Visually significant haze may respond to topical steroids. Recent anecdotal reports indicate that topical difluprednol can be effective in haze reduction, although there are no peer-reviewed articles in the literature at this time regarding the efficacy of topical difluprednate for corneal haze following surface ablation.

Persistent haze may be treated with débridement with intraoperative mitomycin C (Figure 10-2). Patients with visually significant haze may have to wait a number of months prior to consideration of retreatment. If topical steroids are used for prolonged periods, intraocular pressures should be monitored regularly.

Night Vision Disturbance

With any refractive excimer treatment, it will generally take longer for night vision symptoms to resolve. Symptoms can include glare, halos, and reduced vision. The majority of patients will recover to preoperative functioning over a number of weeks to months. A minority of patients may have permanent night vision effects following surface ablation. Reports in the literature are variable regarding the percentage of patients that report persistent night vision disturbances following surface ablation.

There has been a large amount of popular press over the years regarding the risk of night vision reduction. Pupil size has been widely discussed, but has not been definitively proven to be a

Figure 10-1. Corneal haze on optical coherence tomography. (A) This shows the appearance of haze at the level of Bowman's layer following PRK. (B) The decrease in the appearance of haze on OCT correlates with improved vision following treatment with topical steroids in the same patient.

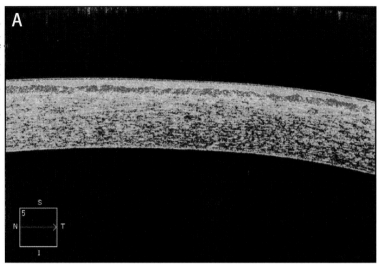

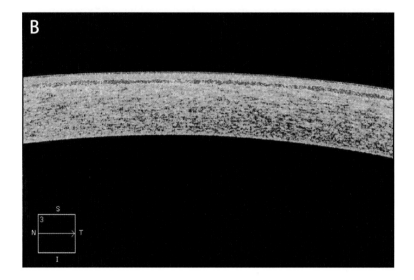

causative factor for night vision complaints following surface ablation (Figure 10-3). Documentation of preoperative night vision complaints can be helpful in documenting baseline.

Patients with visually demanding occupations, such as pilots, paramedics, police, firefighters, and professional divers who do not have control over lighting and may be required to work under low light conditions, should be advised that they may need additional time off or modified shifts. The majority of patients will return to preoperative functioning under low light conditions.

In some cases, residual refractive error can contribute to night vision complaints. Enhancement or prescription glasses for night driving can be helpful in these cases. Pharmacologic pupil constriction has been tried over the years with topical medications including brimonidine, which has a mild miotic effect; however, it is not reliably helpful symptomatically. Some patients find that a lightly yellow-tinted lens enhances contrast at night. While patients may report night vision disturbances, the majority of patients report overall satisfaction with their outcomes from surface ablation.

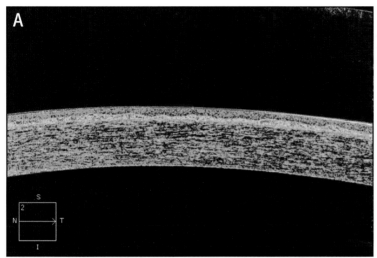

Figure 10-2. Corneal haze before and after treatment with mechanical débridement followed by laser ablation and intraoperative mitomycin.

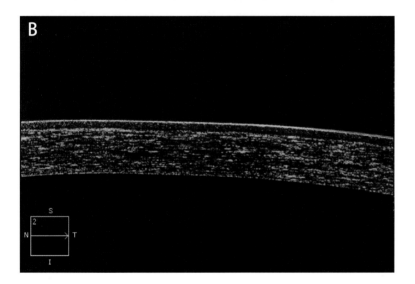

SUMMARY

Complications following surface ablation are uncommon and rarely result in permanent vision loss. However, complications can delay healing or require additional treatment. It is important for prospective patients to know that while the risk is low, it is never possible to guarantee a successful result. Fortunately, the vast majority of surface ablation patients will have an uneventful postoperative course with a high level of satisfaction with the outcome of surgery.

REFERENCES

1. Edmison DR. Lamellar or surface ablation? *J Cataract Refract Surg.* 2003;29(5):858; author reply 858.
2. Khalifa YM, Mifflin MD. Keratitis and corneal melt with ketorolac tromethamine after conductive keratoplasty. *Cornea.* 2011;30(4):477-478.
3. McGee HT, Fraunfelder FW. Toxicities of topical ophthalmic anesthetics. *Expert Opin Drug Saf.* 2007;6(6):637-640.

Figure 10-3. Large pupils can correlate with persistent night vision symptoms following surface ablation, although there are patients with large pupils who do not experience worsening of night vision, and there are some patients with average pupil sizes who complain of increased glare or halo postoperatively.

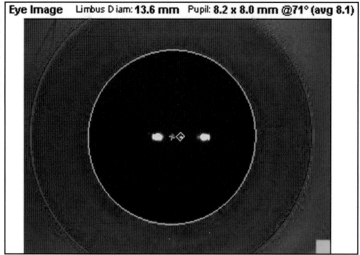

4. de Rojas V, Llovet F, Martínez M, et al. Infectious keratitis in 18,651 laser surface ablation procedures. *J Cataract Refract Surg.* 2011;37(10):1822-1831.
5. Fantes FE, Hanna KD, Waring GO III, Pouliquen Y, Thompson KP, Savoldelli M. Wound healing after excimer laser keratomileusis (photorefractive keratectomy) in monkeys. *Arch Ophthalmol.* 1990;108(5):665-675.
6. Netto MV, Mohan RR, Ambrósio R Jr, Hutcheon AE, Zieske JD, Wilson SE. Wound healing in the cornea: a review of refractive surgery complications and new prospects for therapy. *Cornea.* 2005;24(5):509-522.

11

Special Cases

Surface ablation has been used in combination with intraocular surgery and following other types of corneal surgery (Table 11-1). As discussed in Chapter 9, the epikeratome is not suitable for retreatments after prior corneal surgery.

CONVERSION TO PHOTOREFRACTIVE KERATECTOMY FOLLOWING UNSUCCESSFUL LASIK OR FEMTOSECOND LASIK ATTEMPT

Photorefractive keratectomy (PRK) has been used as an intraoperative alternative over the years for unsuccessful laser-assisted in situ keratomileusis (LASIK) cases where loss of suction occurs. More recent reports involve the use of PRK for failed femtosecond LASIK attempts. This technique is appropriate only when no flap was created but epithelial disruption results.

SURFACE ABLATION FOLLOWING LASIK

PRK for enhancement of uncomplicated LASIK has become more common as patients may present many years after primary surgery for simple retreatment. With stable refraction and normal topography, alcohol-assisted PRK is a common recommended technique for epithelial removal. Corneal brush and epikeratome methods may pose a risk for flap shift or irregular astigmatism.

Complicated LASIK flaps may also be treated with surface ablation.[1,2] For cases with irregular astigmatism, phototherapeutic keratectomy (PTK) or transepithelial PRK may be more appropriate. Successful outcomes have been reported for retreatment of buttonhole, microstriae, and partial flaps (Table 11-2).

Due to the risk of haze, mitomycin C is applied intraoperatively by most surgeons in all cases of surface ablation over a LASIK flap.

Anderson Penno EE. *Surface Ablation: Techniques for Optimum Results (pp 127-133).* © 2013 SLACK Incorporated.

TABLE 11-1. COMBINED SURFACE ABLATION	
Surface ablation has been used following these procedures: • Femtosecond LASIK • LASIK • RK	• IOL implantation • Phakic IOL • Descemet's stripping endothelial keratoplasty • Cross-linking

TABLE 11-2. SURFACE ABLATION FOLLOWING LASIK FLAP COMPLICATIONS	
Surface ablation has been used after LASIK to treat the following: • Microstriae	• Buttonhole • Partial flap • Late enhancement

SURFACE ABLATION FOLLOWING RADIAL KERATOTOMY

PRK and PTK have been used following radial keratotomy (RK). As with any prior corneal surgery, alcohol-assisted PRK or PTK may be the most appropriate method for epithelial removal. RK results in epithelial plugs at the incision sites, which may require additional attention. Wavefront-guided ablations have been reported with good results for PRK following RK.

Diurnal refractive fluctuations and long-term hyperopic shifts can be problematic for retreatment following RK. Instability post-RK makes surgical planning difficult and may impact results following retreatment. Intraoperative mitomycin C is also generally recommended for surface ablation following RK.

The epithelium can be removed using an alcohol-assisted technique. Careful attention should be paid to removing epithelial plugs that may be present at incision sites. Transepithelial surface ablation and wavefront-guided ablation have also been reported.[3,4] Diurnal fluctuations may persist following retreatment after RK.

SURFACE ABLATION FOLLOWING INTRAOCULAR LENS IMPLANTATION

Intentional combination of intraocular and corneal surface techniques to optimize final outcome has been called bioptics. Surface ablation can be used effectively as a planned procedure or as a technique to treat unplanned residual refractive error following intraocular lens (IOL) implantation. With the rising expectations of cataract surgery patients and for refractive lensectomy, even a small amount of residual refractive error can be problematic.

For monofocal IOL implants, a small amount of astigmatism is often well-tolerated. In contrast, for multifocal implants, residual astigmatism can result in significant dissatisfaction. In cases with a normal corneal surface, surface ablation techniques can be effective in achieving emmetropia. There is some debate about the use of wavefront-guided ablation following multifocal IOL due to possible aberrations induced by the IOL.

For standard IOL implants, surface ablation can be helpful in cases of unexpected hyperopia or myopia.

SURFACE ABLATION FOLLOWING PHAKIC INTRAOCULAR LENS IMPLANTATION

Phakic IOL implantation is a smaller but important segment of refractive surgery practice. Recently, there have been reports that, for higher corrections, phakic IOLs may offer a higher quality of vision under mesopic conditions. LASIK has been reported as a combined bioptics technique with phakic IOLs. Some surgeons create a corneal flap prior to phakic IOL implantation in order to reduce risks that may result from the use of a suction ring following lens implantation.

Surface ablation is a suitable alternative for treatment of residual refractive error following phakic IOL implantation. With the exception of epi-LASIK, surface ablation will avoid the potential risks of the suction ring in patients with a phakic IOL. Refractive stability must be confirmed and endothelial cell counts must be obtained prior to considering surface ablation following phakic IOL implantation.

This combined approach, called bioptics, is particularly beneficial for high corrections that may not be suitable for surface ablation. A combined approach may reduce the risks for glare, halo, or reduced night vision in high corrections.

SURFACE ABLATION FOLLOWING DESCEMET'S STRIPPING ENDOTHELIAL KERATOPLASTY

PRK has been reported to be an effective treatment for refractive error following Descemet's stripping endothelial keratoplasty.[5,6]

SURFACE ABLATION IN THIN CORNEAS

As discussed in Chapters 2 and 3, corneal pachymetry and residual stromal bed have been debated for years with respect to the risk of ectasia following corneal laser ablation. Ectasia has been reported more frequently following LASIK but can occur following PRK. Some studies indicate that surface ablation may be safe in thin corneas with normal topography.[7]

SUSPICIOUS OR ABNORMAL TOPOGRAPHY

Abnormal topography is reported as a risk for ectasia following both surface ablation and LASIK.[8] Ectasia risk is discussed in more detail in Chapter 2. In recent years, keratoconus detection software has aided in the detection of abnormal patterns that meet criteria to be considered forme fruste keratoconus.

As discussed in Chapter 2, there are factors including dry eye and contact lens-induced warpage that can cause topographic disturbances. Treatment of dry eye and a longer time out of contact lenses may result in normalization of the topography. Patients with persistent topographic abnormalities that do not meet criteria for forme fruste keratoconus should be approached cautiously when considering surface ablation.

The advent of corneal cross-linking is changing practice patterns for treatment of patients with abnormal topography as discussed next.

Surface Ablation and Cross-Linking

There are increasing numbers of reports of corneal cross-linking for the treatment of keratoconus and ectasia as discussed in Chapter 1 and, in some cases, surface ablation is being combined with intrastromal corneal ring segments and corneal cross-linking. More recently, the prophylactic use of corneal cross-linking has been reported.

It is possible that cross-linking could become standard practice much in the way that mitomycin C use has expanded for some surgeons for use in all cases. As this is a relatively new technique, it may take some time and more prospective studies to determine if cross-linking should be performed as a routine step in refractive laser ablation.

Conductive Keratoplasty Following Photorefractive Keratectomy

Conductive keratoplasty has recently been reported as a method to treat residual refractive error following surface ablation.[9,10]

Summary

Surface ablation is a versatile technique that has been applied to a wide variety of clinical problems with successful outcomes over many years. This versatility is another factor that will keep surface ablation firmly in place as an important tool for refractive surgeons for decades to come.

References

1. Shaikh NM, Wee CE, Kaufman SC. The safety and efficacy of photorefractive keratectomy after laser in situ keratomileusis. *J Refract Surg.* 2005;21(4):353-358.
2. Jain VK, Abell TG, Bond WI, Stevens G Jr. Immediate transepithelial photorefractive keratectomy for treatment of laser in situ keratomileusis flap complications. *J Refract Surg.* 2002;18(2):109-112.
3. Camellin M, Arba Mosquera S. Simultaneous aspheric wavefront-guided transepithelial photorefractive keratectomy and phototherapeutic keratectomy to correct aberrations and refractive errors after corneal surgery. *J Cataract Refract Surg.* 2010;36(7):1173-1180.
4. Ghanem RC, Ghanem VC, Ghanem EA, Kara-José N. Corneal wavefront-guided photorefractive keratectomy with mitomycin-C for hyperopia after radial keratotomy: two-year follow-up. *J Cataract Refract Surg.* 2012;38(4):595-606.
5. Prince J, Chuck RS. Photorefractive keratectomy after Descemet's stripping endothelial keratoplasty. *Curr Opin Ophthalmol.* 2012;23(4):242-245.
6. Awdeh RM, Abbey AM, Vroman DT, et al. Phototherapeutic keratectomy for the treatment of subepithelial fibrosis and anterior corneal scarring after descemet stripping automated endothelial keratoplasty. *Cornea.* 2012;31(7):761-763.
7. Kymionis GD, Bouzoukis D, Diakonis V, et al. Long-term results of thin corneas after refractive laser surgery. *Am J Ophthalmol.* 2007;144(2):181-185.
8. Reznik J, Salz JJ, Klimava A. Development of unilateral corneal ectasia after PRK with ipsilateral preoperative forme fruste keratoconus. *J Refract Surg.* 2008;24(8):843-847.
9. Habibollahi A, Hashemi H, Mehravaran S, Khabazkhoob M. Visual outcomes of conductive keratoplasty to treat hyperopia and astigmatism after laser in situ keratomileusis and photorefractive keratectomy. *Middle East Afr J Ophthalmol.* 2011;18(3):238-242.
10. Hersh PS, Fry KL, Chandrashekhar R, Fikaris DS. Conductive keratoplasty to treat complications of LASIK and photorefractive keratectomy. *Ophthalmology.* 2005;112(11):1941-1947.

SIMULTANEOUS COLLAGEN CROSS-LINKING WITH PHOTOREFRACTIVE KERATECTOMY OR INTRALASE LASIK

Howard V. Gimbel, MD, MPH, FRCSC, FACS and David P. Chan, MD

Laser-assisted in situ keratomileusis (LASIK) and photorefractive keratectomy (PRK) have been recognized to cause weakening of the structural integrity of the cornea by 14% to 33%.[1-4] As a result, iatrogenic ectasia after laser refractive corneal surgery has become a troublesome and unpredictable problem for many corneal refractive surgeons and patients. With the increasing number of eyes undergoing LASIK and PRK, there may be a corresponding increase in the number of corneas that will suffer mechanical fatigue resulting in ectasia.

Corneal cross-linking with riboflavin, generally known as CXL, was first used in 1998 to treat keratoconus.[2] It has been investigated extensively and has been shown clinically to arrest the progression of post-LASIK ectasia as well as keratoconic ectasia.[2-11] With its minimal cost and simplicity and with proven positive clinical outcomes, corneal cross-linking can be regarded as a useful approach to reduce the incidence of postlaser corneal refractive surgery ectasia. The use of CXL has gradually increased and there are currently more than 400 centers around the world performing this procedure.

CXL may also be considered for prophylactic use at the time of corneal refractive surgery because virtually any patient can be treated with cross-linking to reduce the chance of future development of the above conditions. Patients with thinner-than-normal corneas, steeper-than-normal corneas, against-the-rule astigmatism, and especially those with slightly irregular corneal astigmatism shown by asymmetry on corneal topography should be considered for CXL at the time of surgery. The ophthalmic community is starting to see the benefits and minimal risks of prophylactic treatment using CXL and this procedure is now beginning to be offered as a stand-alone procedure or in conjunction with corneal laser refractive surgery (PRK and LASIK). Recent advances in ultraviolet (UV) delivery systems have made it possible to reduce the CXL time to a few minutes. This has increased the practicality of the use of CXL at the time of PRK and LASIK to strengthen the surgically weakened normal cornea and extend the use of these refractive procedures to marginally thin or somewhat asymmetrical corneas. Prophylactic CXL during PRK and LASIK surgery has the added efficiency of being able to apply the riboflavin when the stroma is already exposed after laser treatment, eliminating the need to remove the epithelium just for the treatment. With the appropriate UV light source and riboflavin formulation, the cornea can be prophylactically cross-linked in just a few minutes at the end of a laser corneal refractive procedure.

There may be a slight corneal flattening effect from CXL that would slightly affect the refractive outcome of a corneal refractive procedure and this will have to be studied with a large database. There appears to also be a beneficial refractive stabilizing effect that may be most apparent in hyperopic LASIK corrections as reported by Kanellopoulos, but not yet published. He found less regression of the correction after hyperopic LASIK in eyes that had CXL than in the contralateral eye that did not have CXL.

THE PROCEDURE

The procedure of prophylactic CXL, in essence, is cross-linking at the conclusion of the corneal refractive surgery laser application. The riboflavin solution is applied for the prescribed time directly to the stromal bed after the PRK or LASIK treatment is complete (Figure 11A-1). After rinsing the riboflavin off of the stroma, the LASIK flap is replaced and the UVA light is applied for the prescribed time. For PRK, the UV light is applied before or after rinsing and before the bandage contact lens is applied. Not rinsing keeps the UVA absorption more anterior in the stroma. The recovery is very much the same for PRK or LASIK. With PRK, the re-epithelialization may take a few hours longer. Only one treatment is required.

With most systems in use for therapeutic cross-linking, there is a 30-minute riboflavin (0.1% in 20% dextran) soak time after the epithelium has been removed and then typically 30 minutes of UVA exposure at a 3 mW/cm^2 irradiance. There are newer systems with higher irradiance and

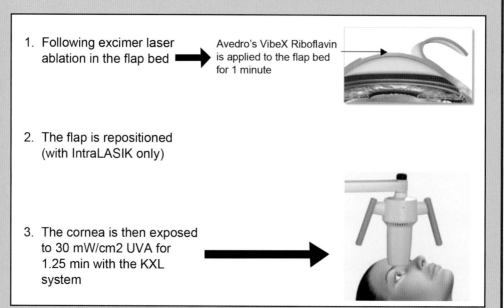

1. Following excimer laser ablation in the flap bed ➡ Avedro's VibeX Riboflavin is applied to the flap bed for 1 minute

2. The flap is repositioned (with IntraLASIK only)

3. The cornea is then exposed to 30 mW/cm2 UVA for 1.25 min with the KXL system

Figure 11A-1. Incorporating cross-linking into intra-LASIK or PRK surgery. (Reprinted with permission from Avedro.)

either flat top or tailored beam profiles. These systems currently have irradiances ranging from 10 to 45 mW/cm². For prophylactic use at the end of PRK or LASIK procedures, different formulations (riboflavin concentrations ranging from 0.1% to 0.25% with and without dextran) are being employed having been CE marked in Europe. Combined soak and UVA illumination times range from 1.5 to 6 minutes using the higher irradiance KXL system, greatly reducing the overall procedure time (Figure 11A-2). These newer protocols have also begun to take into account variation in flap and residual bed thickness. After the flap is closed, the riboflavin diffuses upward into the flap. This acts as a greater riboflavin-absorbing shield. Additional riboflavin soak time and UVA illumination are added to achieve the appropriate amount of UVA absorption of riboflavin in the residual bed.

DISCUSSION

Current studies have shown that CXL is a safe and effective alternative in the treatment of keratoconus, forme fruste keratoconus, pellucid marginal degeneration, and postlaser refractive surgery ectasia.[12-17] More than a decade of results have shown that therapeutic cross-linking appears to last for a long time and there is evidence that the strengthening effect will be permanent. Long-term evaluations will have to be done to determine longer-term efficacy.

For prophylactic use, virtually any corneal excimer laser refractive surgery patient can be treated with cross-linking to reduce the possibility of ectasia development. After PRK and even after LASIK, where one has created a flap of tissue on the cornea and then removed some stromal tissue, the structural strength of the cornea is stronger after the procedure than before when using prophylactic CXL. It is still possible to perform LASIK or PRK enhancement after CXL with riboflavin. Also, CXL treatment can be repeated if necessary.

Prophylactic CXL may extend the parameters for safe corneal refractive surgery. Some patients with thinner-than-normal corneas, asymmetry on corneal topography, against-the-rule astigmatism, or steeper-than-normal corneas that have been counseled against laser corneal refractive surgery may now qualify if combined with CXL.

Curently, those patients who do not qualify for CXL include pregnant or nursing women and those with riboflavin allergy, a history of herpes infection or chemical corneal injury, concurrent eye infection, aphakia, pseudophakia with an IOL that does not block UV light, corneal thickness of less than 375 μm (less than 325 μm with VibeX Rapid [Avedro, Waltham, MA]), history of poor epithelial

PRK Xtra/IntraLASIK Xtra

- Efficacy: strengthens cornea by 4x
- Speed: 75-second UVA exposure with high power (3 mW/cm^2 versus 30 mW/cm^2)
- Safety: 1-minute soak time—IntraLASIK
    3-minute soak time—PRK
- Predictability: uniform beam profile (consistent energy delivered across the cornea)

Figure 11A-2. Summary of riboflavin soak and UV exposure times. (Reprinted with permission from Avedro.)

wound healing, autoimmune disease, nystagmus, and those taking vitamin C supplements within 1 week before treatment (vitamin C decreases the UVA absorption of riboflavin).

REFERENCES

1. Ali Javadi M, Kanavi MR, Mahdavi M, et al. Comparison of keratocyte density between keratoconus, post-laser in situ keratomileusis keratectasia, and uncomplicated post-laser in situ keratomileusis. *Cornea.* 2009;28(7):774-779.
2. Wollensak G, Spoerl E, Seiler T. Riboflavin/ultraviolet-A-induced collagen crosslinking for the treatment of keratoconus. *Am J Ophthalmol.* 2003;135(5):620-627.
3. Wollensak G. Crosslinking treatment of progressive keratoconus: new hope. *Curr Opin Ophthalmol.* 2006;17(4):356-360.
4. Hafezi F, Kanellopoulos J, Wiltfang R, Seiler T. Corneal collagen crosslinking with riboflavin and ultraviolet A to treat induced keratectasia after laser in situ keratomileusis. *J Cataract Refract Surg.* 2007;33(12):2035-2040.
5. Spadea L. Corneal collagen cross-linking with riboflavin and UVA irradiation in pellucid marginal degeneration. *J Refract Surg.* 2010;26(5):375-377.
6. Raiskup-Wolf F, Hoyer A, Spoerl E, Pillunat LE. Collagen crosslinking with riboflavin and ultraviolet-A light in keratoconus: long-term results. *J Cataract Refract Surg.* 2008;34(5):796-801.
7. Coskunseven E, Jankov MR 2nd, Hafezi F. Contralateral eye study of corneal collagen cross-linking with riboflavin and UVA irradiation in patients with keratoconus. *J Refract Surg.* 2009;25(4):371-376.
8. Vinciguerra P, Albè E, Trazza S, et al. Refractive, topographic, tomographic, and aberrometric analysis of keratoconic eyes undergoing corneal cross-linking. *Ophthalmology.* 2009;116(3):369-378.
9. Caporossi A, Mazzotta C, Baiocchi S, Caporossi T. Long-term results of riboflavin ultraviolet A corneal collagen cross-linking for keratoconus in Italy: the Siena Eye Cross Study. *Am J Ophthalmol.* 2010;149(4):585-593.
10. Kymionis GD. Corneal collagen cross-linking—PLUS. *Open Ophthalmol J.* 2011;5:10.
11. Kanellopoulos AJ, Binder PS. Collagen cross-linking (CCL) with sequential topography-guided PRK: a temporizing alternative for keratoconus to penetrating keratoplasty. *Cornea.* 2007;26(7):891-895.
12. Kymionis GD, Karavitaki AE, Kounis GA, Portaliou DM, Yoo SH, Pallikaris IG. Management of pellucid marginal corneal degeneration with simultaneous customized photorefractive keratectomy and collagen crosslinking. *J Cataract Refract Surg.* 2009;35(7):1298-1301.
13. Kymionis GD, Kontadakis GA, Kounis GA, et al. Simultaneous topography-guided PRK followed by corneal collagen cross-linking for keratoconus. *J Refract Surg.* 2009;25(9):S807-S811.
14. Kanellopoulos AJ. Comparison of sequential vs same-day simultaneous collagen cross-linking and topographyguided PRK for treatment of keratoconus. *J Refract Surg.* 2009;25(9):S812-S818.
15. Stojanovic A, Zhang J, Chen X, Nitter TA, Chen S, Wang Q. Topography-guided transepithelial surface ablation followed by corneal collagen cross-linking performed in a single combined procedure for the treatment of keratoconus and pellucid marginal degeneration. *J Refract Surg.* 2010;26(2):145-152.
16. Kymionis GD, Portaliou DM, Kounis GA, Limnopoulou AN, Kontadakis GA, Grentzelos MA. Simultaneous topography-guided photorefractive keratectomy followed by corneal collagen cross-linking for keratoconus. *Am J Ophthalmol.* 2011;152(5):748-755.
17. Tuwairqi WS, Sinjab MM. Safety and efficacy of simultaneous corneal collagen cross-linking with topography-guided PRK in managing low-grade keratoconus: 1-year follow-up. *J Refract Surg.* 2012;28(5):341-345.

12

Factors Affecting Patient Satisfaction

Every refractive surgeon has observed the variability in patient satisfaction with some patients very satisfied with some residual refractive error and some patients unhappy with excellent uncorrected distance vision. While it is not possible to guarantee satisfaction, there are several factors that can influence postoperative satisfaction. As outlined in Chapter 3, these can include expectations as well as outcomes. There is some indication that depression might be a risk factor for dissatisfaction following excimer laser surgery.

There has been increasing interest in studying patient satisfaction in recent years.[1] With more than a million corneal refractive surgery procedures performed each year in the United States alone, even a low complication rate can result in a substantial number of people who may be unhappy with their results. Due to increasing complaints, the US Food and Drug Administration (FDA) launched the "LASIK Quality of Life Project" in 2009 in order to study the impact of refractive surgery on perceived quality of life.

FOOD AND DRUG ADMINISTRATION LASIK QUALITY OF LIFE PROJECT

The LASIK Quality of Life Project is jointly funded by the FDA, the National Eye Institute (NEI), and the US Department of Defense. The stated aim of the project is to identify factors that can affect quality of life after laser-assisted in situ keratomileusis (LASIK) and to potentially reduce adverse effects that can affect outcomes. In 2009, when the project was launched, the FDA also sent warning letters to surgery centers that were not complying with earlier legislation requiring surgery centers to report deaths or adverse events relating to surgical devices.

The project will have 3 phases. In phase one, an online questionnaire is to be developed to evaluate quality-of-life issues and outcomes reported by patients following LASIK. The second phase will evaluate outcomes and quality-of-life issues in a population of active-duty patients treated at the Navy Refractive Surgery Center at the Navy Medical Center in San Diego. Phase three is to undertake a multicenter national clinical trial to assess outcomes and quality-of-life issues following LASIK in the general population.

Although the study specifically mentions LASIK, it is likely that there will be important information collected regarding surface ablation as a comparative treatment.

Anderson Penno EE. *Surface Ablation: Techniques for Optimum Results* (pp 135-140).
© 2013 SLACK Incorporated.

TABLE 12-1. MOST COMMON REASONS FOR DISSATISFACTION
• Decreased uncorrected visual acuity due to regression or residual refractive error
• Dry eye
• Poor vision in dim lighting
• Night halos
• Older age

WHAT IS SATISFACTION?

Most studies report best-corrected visual acuity (BCVA) and refractive error. Some include night vision disturbance and dry eye. These are all important outcomes but will not necessarily predict patient satisfaction. A patient will be most satisfied when his or her expectations are met or exceeded. A practice of under-promising and over-delivering will help improve overall patient satisfaction. As discussed in Chapter 3, setting appropriate expectations is critical, but sometimes difficult in the face of aggressive marketing campaigns giving guarantees or your money back or promising better vision than is possible with corrective lenses.

The NEI has developed an online questionnaire called the NEI Refractive Error Quality of Life Instrument-42 (NEI RQL-42) that is available at www.nei.nih.gov/resources/pdfs/nei-rql-42-1.pdf and has been used to study quality of life following refractive surgery. A recent study using this questionnaire reported that as compared the emmetropes, LASIK patients perceived a -7.1% quality of life, ortho-keratography patients -13%, spectacle wearers -15.8%, and soft contact lens patients a -17.3% reduction in quality-of-life scores.[2] In the future, a standardized tool such as the NEI RQL-42 would be useful in comparing surface ablation techniques to each other and to other types of vision correction.

A recent large meta-analysis of LASIK satisfaction articles found that the timing of the questionnaire affected the results.[1] Studies completed within the first 6 months postoperatively reported that an average of 94.8% of patients were satisfied with their outcome. This average rose to 98.5% for studies conducted at or later than 7 months postoperatively. It is most likely that this would be even more dramatic with postsurface ablation patients due to the nature of the corneal surface remodeling that occurs following no-flap treatments. This difference can be mitigated by pre- and postoperative counseling.

Most common reasons for dissatisfaction included decreased uncorrected visual acuity (UCVA) due to residual refractive error or regression, dry eye, decreased scotopic vision, night halos, and older age (Table 12-1). As mentioned in Chapter 3, depressive symptoms preoperatively are correlated with more dissatisfaction after refractive surgery. Satisfaction and quality-of-life issues may vary from patient to patient. As most refractive surgeons know, postoperative visual acuity does not predict satisfaction.

EXPECTATIONS

Careful preoperative counseling can avoid unhappy postoperative patients (see Table 12-1). This is the most important step in improving postoperative dissatisfaction as discussed in Chapter 3. Taking time before surgery to be sure that patients understand healing time and final outcome expectations can save time postoperatively if expectations are not met. Patients may think they are informed well enough by their friends or their Internet surfing, but the only way to be sure is to have a systematic patient education routine as part of your practice.

TABLE 12-2. COMMON MOTIVATIONS FOR SURFACE ABLATION	
• Convenience	• Occupation
• Safety	• Health
• Self-confidence	• Comfort*
• Financial	• Improved vision*
*These may be red flags for unrealistic expectations.	

Unhappy 20/20 patients often have inappropriate expectations, such as not understanding that, if they are presbyopic, they will need reading glasses. The mild myope who takes glasses off to read may not understand that correcting for distance will take away their uncorrected near vision. Another frequent cause for dissatisfaction is the misconception that refractive surgery will correct dry eye because it eliminates the need for contact lenses.

It is critical for surface ablation patients to understand the time it takes for recovery of their best vision.[3] Most patients are understanding of the first few days with a bandage contact lens in place; however, many patients will expect that their vision will be as sharp as it was with corrective lenses preoperatively as soon as the contacts are removed. Some patients will have trips, new jobs, weddings, or other important events planned within a week of surgery.

It is important to tell surface ablation patients that they may experience some fluctuations, night vision symptoms, dry eye, ghosting, or blurred vision for weeks or sometimes months following surgery. This is particularly important for surface ablation patients who may have friends or family members who have had LASIK.

Document that the patient has read the informed consent and watched an educational video if provided. If the patient has not read the consent prior to surgery, take the extra time to have the patient read it before proceeding with a preoperative sedative. Although complications are uncommon with surface ablation, the risk is not zero and patients must accept there is some risk to any refractive surgery treatment.

Presbyopic patients may benefit from a monovision contact lens trial or showing full correction in a trial frame with a reading card. In some cases, declining to accept a patient for surgery due to inappropriate expectations may be the right choice.

It is helpful to understand the patient's motivations to undergo surface ablation.[4] Commonly stated reasons are summarized in Table 12-2. Many surgeons will have heard stories such as the moderate myope who had her glasses knocked off during a car accident and after experiencing the panic of being in a chaotic situation and unable to see properly, decided to have refractive surgery. Other patients will have financial reasons for having surgery due to the estimated costs of glasses or contact lenses over time compared to the one-time surgery fee.

Using tools such as telephone screening questionnaires, written patient education materials, educational DVDs or videos, and checklists for patient counseling can help standardize the process (Table 12-3). Good communication skills are an asset for both surgeon and staff as well.[5] With all these tools, unrealistic expectations can often be identified, and the majority of patients will have appropriate expectations for surgical outcome.

RESIDUAL REFRACTIVE ERROR

Refractive error is a common reason for complaints of blurred vision and may contribute to night vision difficulties. In some cases, enhancement might be appropriate if refraction is stable. If

TABLE 12-3. TOOLS FOR SETTING APPROPRIATE EXPECTATIONS

- Telephone screening questionnaires for inquiries and booking
- Written patient educational materials
- Educational DVDs/videos
- Good communication skills

the refraction becomes unstable years following surface ablation, then other disorders such as diabetes or cataract should be considered. Depending on the individual patient, prescription glasses for occasional use such as night driving can be helpful. If enhancement is not recommended due to unstable refraction or other reasons, taking time to discuss these reasons with the patient can lead to better overall satisfaction.

PRESBYOPIA

In spite of excellent preoperative counseling, some presbyopic patients are still disappointed with their near vision following surface ablation for distance. Cycloplegic refraction should be considered for all patients who are dissatisfied with acuity following surface ablation. In some cases, there may be latent hyperopia due to over-response from myopic correction or under-response for a hyperopic correction. For these cases, enhancement may be considered, particularly if the dominant eye is affected and if the patient is complaining about distance blur.

With the advent of presbyopic laser ablation patterns, there will likely be an increased number of patients who may have the expectation that they will be free from reading glasses. A key to satisfaction for presbyopic treatments will be to provide the appropriate expectation. For monovision, a contact lens trial provides an excellent learning tool for the patient to understand what the intended outcome will provide in terms of visual functioning.

DRY EYE

Dry eye is common both before and after refractive surgery. Again, in spite of careful preoperative counseling, some patients believe that if they have contact lenses, refractive surgery will eliminate dry eye by eliminating the need for contacts. Patients who wear glasses may have a permanently drier eye due to the fact their eyes are more exposed following surface ablation.

Managing persistent dry eye postoperatively will often involve several visits over a number of months. Most patients will need some combination of treatment with lubricants, lid care, and in some cases, antihistamine drops. Topical cyclosporine may be helpful for dry eye that persists longer than 3 to 6 months.

Punctal plugs can help in some patients, although active patients may notice tearing with outdoor activities. Punctal plugs do not eliminate the need to treat coexisting disorders, such as blepharitis and allergies. Some patients are frustrated by the chronic nature of ocular surface disease and the need for ongoing management.

NIGHT VISION

Night vision will take longer to improve following surface ablation than vision in brighter light. Supporting patients during this period with counseling, modification of work schedules, or additional time off work will lead to higher satisfaction. As with other potential side effects of surface ablation, some patients will be surprised by glare or halo at night even if they had been warned of the possibility.

High corrections and larger pupils have been discussed as possible risk factors for night vision disturbance following excimer refractive surgery, but it can be difficult to predict which patients will have more difficulty at night. Pupil size has never been definitively proven to result in permanent night vision effects. Documenting night vision concerns prior to surgery will also help to determine whether these effects were present prior to surgery.

Enhancement may be helpful when appropriate or night driving glasses may help in some cases. Anecdotally, patients will sometimes complain about red LED displays causing persistent glare, which may or may not resolve.

LOSS OF BEST-CORRECTED VISUAL ACUITY

In spite of careful preoperative screening, complications can occur. Fortunately, loss of best-corrected visual acuity (BCVA) is uncommon following surface ablation but it has been reported. Rare events such as severe infection, ectasia, visually significant haze, or steroid-induced ocular hypertension can result in permanent vision loss.

It is the success of excimer refractive surgery over many years that has led the general public to have high expectations of safety. With the goal of minimizing risks through surface ablation, attention to details such as predisposing risk factors before surgery and careful monitoring for signs of infection and elevated intraocular pressure postoperatively can be effective. Consents should include rare but sight-threatening potential complications.

MANAGEMENT OF UNHAPPY PATIENTS

Maintaining a good rapport with patients prior to and during surgery will lay groundwork for management of complications or cases where the patient has a good outcome but had inappropriate expectations. Resist the urge to avoid unhappy patients and do not get pressured into retreatment when it may be too early or has a low likelihood of improving BCVA or quality of vision.

Surgeons may feel they want to avoid the unhappy patient; however, these patients should be given more time rather than less (Table 12-4). Provide additional appointments to discuss concerns, follow up with telephone calls, and complete supportive documentation where needed for work duties or insurance.

Book extra time for appointments and sit while listening to the patients' concerns. Sitting and facing a patient during a discussion will reassure the patient that you are in fact paying attention to his or her concerns. Refer back to preoperative notes if helpful to remind the patient of expectations that were discussed preoperatively (such as readers). Remember that 20/20 does not measure comfort or quality of vision.

Remedies, if available, should be discussed. Although the goal of surface ablation is to reduce dependence on corrective lenses, glasses or contact lenses may be helpful for some cases in which further surgery is not advisable. If further recovery is expected, such as in dry eye, support the patient during the time required for treatments such as topical cyclosporine A.

TABLE 12-4. TOOLS FOR MANAGING DISSATISFACTION

- Allowing for extra time for appointments
- Sitting face-to-face while talking to the patient
- Scheduling time with the surgeon
- Arranging for second opinion
- Providing documentation support for time of work or other forms
- Consulting with risk-management professionals
- Discussing possible remedies such as glasses, contact lenses, or other treatments if applicable
- Referring to prior documentation regarding expected results and possible risks

Second opinions can be helpful for both the surgeon and patient in particularly difficult cases. Document all interactions including telephone calls. Contact risk management professionals for additional support.

SUMMARY

With the recent increase in interest in quality-of-life issues, refractive surgeons will likely have better tools in the future to identify preoperative factors that may be a risk for dissatisfaction following surgery.

REFERENCES

1. Solomon KD, Fernández de Castro LE, Sandoval HP, et al, Joint LASIK Study Task Force. LASIK world literature review: quality of life and patient satisfaction. *Ophthalmology.* 2009;116(4):691-701.
2. Queirós A, Villa-Collar C, Gutiérrez AR, Jorge J, González-Méijome JM. Quality of life of myopic subjects with different methods of visual correction using the NEI RQL-42 questionnaire. *Eye Contact Lens.* 2012;38(2):116-121.
3. Manche EE, Haw WW. Wavefront-guided laser in situ keratomileusis (Lasik) versus wavefront-guided photorefractive keratectomy (Prk): a prospective randomized eye-to-eye comparison (an American Ophthalmological Society thesis). *Trans Am Ophthalmol Soc.* 2011;109:201-220.
4. Packer M. Do you know your patient's goal? *Curr Opin Ophthalmol.* 2009;20(1):1-2.
5. Lin DJ, Sheu IC, Pai JY, et al. Measuring patients' expectations and the perception of quality in LASIK services. *Health Qual Life Outcomes.* 2009;7:63.

Conclusion

Surface ablation is deceptively simple in terms of surgical technique but requires an in-depth knowledge of individual patient characteristics, including psychological factors such as expectations along with the technical knowledge of diagnosis, treatment, and wound healing following treatment. There are numerous factors that will influence outcomes and satisfaction following surface ablation. For successful refractive outcomes, the surgeon needs to be attentive to all steps in the process.

Patient selection is the first step on the road to optimal results. As outlined in this book, there are a large number of factors that need to be considered before determining if the patient will be likely to have an acceptably low risk and positive outcome from surface ablation. Standardized checklists can be a good tool to ensure a thorough approach to preoperative assessment.

If the surgeon can do the assessment, it can streamline the assessment process by allowing for additional testing to be performed at that time. Surgeon assessment also avoids having to cancel a patient on the day of surgery, which can be upsetting to the patient and stressful for the surgeon.

The second step for a successful outcome is patient education. An educated patient is more likely to have appropriate expectations as well as an understanding of the possible risks—although low, the risks are real. In this era of medicine-meets-retail advertising, many patients may have the misconception that it is possible to provide 100% safety and guarantee results. It is not possible and can be a disaster to over-promise results of surface ablation even with the latest technology.

The third step in the process is to provide excellent service with efficient staff and a standardized surgical approach. There are an astonishing number of factors that can affect outcomes, including individual corneal biomechanics, wound healing, patient psychological issues such as expectations or anxiety, laser type, surgical technique, and excimer platform. By using a standard approach and a specific array of techniques, a surgeon can discern factors that, in their experience, may lead to adverse outcomes or that can lead to improved outcomes.

The final step is to provide caring postoperative service. This is of particular importance in the first days and weeks following surface ablation. Many patients are expecting the first few days to be the most difficult but underestimate the longer-term healing that can occur in the first months following surface ablation.

Corneal refractive surgery continues to evolve and improve. It is as exciting a time to provide refractive surgery as it was a quarter century ago when the excimer laser was first introduced. It is impossible to predict what the next decade will bring but it is sure to lead to better outcomes and improved satisfaction for refractive surgery patients. Surface ablation is likely to remain a part of the refractive landscape for the foreseeable future.

Anderson Penno EE. *Surface Ablation:*
Techniques for Optimum Results (p 141).
© 2013 SLACK Incorporated.

Appendix

SAMPLE COMANAGEMENT AND EDUCATIONAL MATERIALS

*All materials should be modified as needed to conform to local medicolegal recommendations.

1. Comanaged Refractive Surgery Referral Form

Referral Date (d/m/yr) _____

Patient Name: _____

Date of Birth: (d/m/yr)_____

A.H.C. # _____

Address: _____

City and State: _____ Postal Code: _____

Phone Numbers: h: _____ w: _____ c:_____

E-mail address:_____

Referring Doctor: _____

Fax Number: _____ **Address:** _____

Phone Number: _____ **E-mail:** _____

Ocular History (ie, previous injury, amblyopia, previous eye surgery, dry eye):_____

_____

_____

Family history of keratoconus or other: _____

_____

Medical Information:

Please report if patient has an autoimmune disease, rheumatoid arthritis, diabetes, ocular herpes zoster or herpes simplex, collagen vascular disease, hepatitis, or is pregnant or nursing:

_____

_____

Please list any medications the patient may be taking:_____

_____

Please list any allergies (nuts, shellfish, medications, surgical tape, latex, eye drops, etc): ____

_____

Does the patient wear prisms in her/his glasses? ❏ Yes   ❏ No
Does the patient wear contact lenses? ❏ Hard   ❏ Soft   ❏ RGP   ❏ Other
VA SC: OD: 20/ OS: 20/

Anderson Penno EE. *Surface Ablation:*
Techniques for Optimum Results (pp 143-153).
© 2013 SLACK Incorporated.

Glasses Rx: OD _____   VA 20/_____
              OS _____   VA 20/_____
Manifest: OD _____   VA 20/_____
              OS _____   VA 20/_____
Cycloplegic: OD _____   VA 20/_____
              OS _____   VA 20/_____
Vertex Distance: Manifest _____ mm   Cycloplegic _____ mm
Keratometry Readings:
       OD: _____@ _____/ _____@ _____
       OS: _____@ _____/ _____@ _____
Intraocular Pressure: _____ NCT   _____ AT   OD: _____ mm Hg   OS: _____ mm Hg
Pupil Reactions: PERRL Other:_____
Pupil Size (diameter in room and dim illumination):
   OD: Room _____ mm   Dim _____ mm
   OS: Room _____ mm   Dim _____ mm
Anterior Segment: OD: Normal/Other _____
                   OS: Normal/Other _____
Posterior Segment: Dilated _____   Undilated _____
C/D ratio: OD _____   OS_____
Macula: OD _____   OS_____
Periphery: OD _____   OS_____
Pachymetry: OD _____   OS_____
Monovision Discussed: ☐ Yes ☐ No
Monovision Trial: ☐ Yes ☐ No
Motivation for Surgery: _____
Summary: _____
_____
_____
_____

2. Refractive Patient Checklist

Patient Name: _____

☐ Call patient 1 to 2 weeks prior to ref assess (contacts out)
☐ Patient (pt) watched DVD
☐ EEP identifies if pt is a candidate for Sx
☐ Given brochures including pricing info
☐ Call if have not heard back from pt
☐ Book repeat Wavescan if over 30 days before Sx
☐ Sx package sent including:
    ☐ Surgery confirmation letter (quote, Sx fees, discounts, comanagement)
    ☐ Preop instructions letter (PRK or LASIK)
    ☐ Consent form (PRK or LASIK)
    ☐ Time off work letter (3 days LASIK, 10 days PRK)
    ☐ Rx for eye drops
☐ Letter to optom if Sx booked
☐ Confirm 1 to 2 weeks prior to Sx (no contacts)
☐ Comanagement fees to optom (if applicable)
☐ Notify Medicare when Sx complete

❏ Postop appts:

PRK	*LASIK*
❏ 1 day postop	❏ 1 day postop
❏ 3 day postop	❏ 1 week postop
❏ 1 week postop	❏ 1 month postop
❏ 1 month postop	❏ 3 month postop
❏ 3 month postop	❏ 6 month postop
❏ 6 month postop	

❏ Letter for driver's license

❏ Keratometry readings to pt

❏ Satisfaction survey sent (3 month after Sx)

3. Patient Information—Epi-LASIK Surgery

Introduction

The excimer laser reshapes the curvature of the cornea to possibly reduce or eliminate the need for glasses or contact lenses in cases of myopia (nearsightedness), hyperopia (farsightedness), and/ or astigmatism.

Epi-LASIK is a procedure that uses an extremely fine and precise instrument called an epi-keratome to cut a thin flap of the epithelium from the surface of the cornea. A suction ring is attached to the eye securing it for the epi-keratome. Most people will describe a feeling of pressure during the procedure. The excimer laser is then used to correct the patient's refractive error.

The epithelial flap is removed, leaving a precise edge with a smooth central zone to which the excimer laser energy is applied. Epi-LASIK has the safety of a no-flap procedure with faster recovery than standard PRK.

How the Eye Works

To better understand epi-LASIK and how the excimer laser can be used to correct vision problems resulting from refractive errors, a short review of how the eye works may be helpful. Refractive errors generally result from an elongated or irregularly shaped eye. When light enters the eye, it is bent (refracted) by a clear, strong tissue at the front of the eye called the cornea. The cornea, in effect, acts like a lens to focus incoming light onto the retina at the back of the eye.

In myopia (nearsightedness), light entering the eye does not focus on the retina as it should; instead, the image is focused at a point in front of the retina. The result is that distant objects appear blurry while objects close to the viewer can be seen in focus. Nearsightedness is frequently caused by either an abnormally long eye or by an excessively steep curvature of the cornea.

In hyperopia (farsightedness), light entering the eye focuses images at a point behind the retina so the image is not focused before it reaches the retina. This is frequently caused by an eye that is abnormally short or by an excessively flat cornea. With farsightedness, close objects appear blurry while objects in the distance can be seen in focus.

In astigmatism, the problem is not in the length of the eye, but the fact that the cornea is not spherical and contains different curvatures. The eye is shaped more like a football than like a soccer ball. The result of astigmatism is that the objects do not focus into a single image and the vision is distorted or blurry. Most of the population has some varying degree of astigmatism.

Presbyopia, or the inability to see close objects, usually becomes apparent to most people in their early to mid-forties. This condition normally occurs with age and results from a change in the eye when the natural lens loses its ability to focus on close objects.

Epi-LASIK, which reshapes only the cornea, cannot be used to correct presbyopia.

Patients Who Wear Contact Lenses

Contact lenses can distort the curvature of the cornea after prolonged use. Therefore, before being evaluated for epi-LASIK and before the treatment can be performed, the shape of the cornea must be allowed to stabilize in its natural shape. Staff will advise you as to the amount of time required to remove your contact lenses prior to surgery.

The Epi-LASIK Procedure

Before proceeding with the epi-LASIK surgery, all your final testing and mapping will be done and reviewed to detect and isolate any irregularities in the health and shape of the corneas. Upon arriving at the laser center, you will be seated in the waiting area. Prior to surgery, antibiotic and anti-inflammatory drops will be administered. If at any time prior to the surgery you have any questions or concerns, our staff will be available to review the procedure with you. Most patients dress casually and comfortably. You are reminded not to wear any eye make-up, cologne, or perfume and to bring a companion to drive you home. Patients are not to drive the day of the surgery.

Treatment

In the laser room, you will be seated in a chair, which reclines and rotates for proper positioning with respect to the laser used to perform epi-LASIK. The eye that is not being treated will be covered with gauze and the chair will be aligned under the laser for the first eye surgery. The eye being treated will receive a topical anesthetic eye drop. The lids and skin surrounding the eye will be cleaned.

Next, an instrument called a lid speculum will be placed between your upper and lower eyelids to prevent you from blinking. The surgeon will then start the epi-LASIK treatment and will apply the suction ring to the eye. When the suction is applied, the vision will appear dimmed or darkened—you will not see or feel the epithelial removal. The flap is made with the epi-keratome and the suction ring is removed. The hinged flap will be lifted and removed, the laser will be activated, and the reshaping of the cornea will begin. The surgeon will put additional medications in the eye to prevent infection and the lid speculum will be removed. Some patients may experience discomfort in the hours following treatment; therefore, appropriate pain-relieving medications will be prescribed.

Total time in the laser room is usually less than 30 minutes if both eyes are being treated.

Postprocedure Expectations

After the surgery, you will be advised to rest for the remainder of the day and to continue using prescribed eye drops as instructed. Before you leave the laser center, you will be supplied with a kit containing antibiotic and anti-inflammatory eye drops and a schedule for their use. Patients return to the office the day following the procedure to confirm that the healing process is progressing satisfactorily.

The staff will monitor your recovery and will advise you on the use of the eye drops. Steroid eye drops are used after the procedure to regulate the healing progress and to reduce redness and eye irritation. In order to achieve optimal results, it is recommended that you follow the drop regimen impeccably. Some patients have developed adverse effects from the topical medications, such as drug allergy or toxicity reactions. Prolonged use of the steroid drops can be associated with cataract production or the development of steroid-induced raised intraocular pressure.

Periodic Tests and Follow-Up

You will be required to undergo certain tests, including vision assessments and other measurements at our office, before and after the procedure. Postoperative exams are scheduled 24 to 48 hours for the first 1 to 5 days to monitor your progress after surgery. Follow-up will then be required at 1 to 2 weeks and then monthly for approximately 3 to 4 months.

If laser enhancement is required, a repeat procedure can be performed once the refraction is stable, which is usually after 6 months.

Financial Responsibility

There will be a charge for each eye depending on your candidacy for conventional treatment or customized treatment. This is the sole responsibility of the patient and must be paid in full prior to the surgery. Retreatments/enhancement surgery(s) are included in the fees for each eye for a time frame of 18 months postoperatively.

Alternate Treatment

You are free to decide not to have this operation. If you decide not to have this procedure for the correction of nearsightedness (myopia), farsightedness (hyperopia), and/or astigmatism, there are other methods of restoring vision without excimer laser surgery, including but not limited to eyeglasses, contact lenses, or other refractive surgeries depending on your ocular health.

4. Patient Information—Photorefractive Keratectomy Surgery

Introduction

The excimer laser reshapes the curvature of the cornea to possibly reduce or eliminate the need for glasses or contact lenses in cases of myopia (nearsightedness), hyperopia (farsightedness), and/or astigmatism. Photorefractive keratectomy (PRK) is an excimer laser procedure that reshapes the corneal curvature.

How the Eye Works

To better understand PRK and how the excimer laser can be used to correct vision problems resulting from refractive errors, a short review of how the eye works may be helpful. Refractive errors generally result from an elongated or irregularly shaped eye. When light enters the eye, it is bent (refracted) by a clear, strong tissue at the front of the eye called the cornea. The cornea, in effect, acts like a lens to focus incoming light onto the retina at the back of the eye.

In myopia (nearsightedness), light entering the eye does not focus on the retina as it should; instead, the image is focused at a point in front of the retina. The result is that distant objects appear blurry while objects near the viewer can be seen in focus. Nearsightedness is frequently caused by either an abnormally long eye or by an excessively steep curvature of the cornea.

In hyperopia (farsightedness), light entering the eye focuses images at a point behind the retina so the image is not focused before it reaches the retina. This is frequently caused by an eye that is abnormally short or by an excessively flat cornea. With farsightedness, close objects appear blurry while objects in the distance can be seen in focus.

In astigmatism, the problem is not in the length of the eye but the fact that the cornea is not spherical and contains different curvatures. The eye is shaped more like a football than like a soccer ball. The result of astigmatism is that the objects do not focus into a single image and the vision is distorted or blurry. Most of the population has some varying degree of astigmatism.

Presbyopia, or the inability to see close objects, usually becomes apparent to most people in their early to mid-forties. This condition occurs normally with age and results from a change in the eye when the natural lens loses its ability to focus on close objects. PRK, which reshapes only the cornea, cannot be used to correct presbyopia.

Patients Who Wear Contact Lenses

Contact lenses can distort the curvature of the cornea after prolonged use. Therefore, before being evaluated for PRK and before the treatment can be performed, the shape of the cornea must be allowed to stabilize in its natural shape. Staff will advise you as to the amount of time required to remove your contact lenses prior to surgery.

The Photorefractive Keratectomy Procedure

Before proceeding with the PRK surgery, all your final testing and mapping will be done and reviewed to detect and isolate any irregularities in the health and shape of the corneas. Upon arriving at the laser center, you will be seated in the waiting area. Prior to surgery, antibiotic and anti-inflammatory drops will be administered. If at any time prior to the surgery you have any questions or concerns, our staff will be available to review the procedure with you. Most patients dress casually and comfortably. You are reminded not to wear any eye make-up, cologne, or per-fume and to bring a companion to drive you home. Patients are not to drive the day of the surgery.

Treatment

In the laser room, you will be seated in a chair that reclines and rotates for proper positioning with respect to the laser used to perform PRK. The eye that is not being treated will be covered with gauze and the chair will be aligned under the laser for the first eye surgery. The eye being treated will receive a topical anesthetic eye drop. The lids and skin surrounding the eye will be cleaned.

Next, an instrument called a lid speculum will be placed between your upper and lower eyelids to prevent you from blinking. You will be asked to focus on a blinking red light. The laser treat-ment pulses will be controlled by the surgeon with a footswitch. During the laser treatment, you will hear a snapping sound and may notice an odor.

You will not feel the laser action. Following the laser, a contact lens will be placed on the cornea. During the hours following the treatment, you may experience discomfort for which you can take drops or oral medications. Medications will be reviewed with you on the day of surgery. Total time in the laser room is usually less than 30 minutes if both eyes are being treated.

Postprocedure Expectations

After the surgery, you will be advised to rest for the remainder of the day and to continue using prescribed eye drops as instructed. Before you leave the laser center, you will be supplied with a kit containing antibiotic and anti-inflammatory eye drops and a schedule for their use. Patients return to the office the day after the procedure to confirm that the healing process is progressing satisfactorily.

The staff will monitor your recovery and will advise you on the use of the eye drops. Steroid eye drops are used after the procedure to regulate the healing progress and to reduce redness and eye irritation. In order to achieve optimal results, it is recommended that you follow the drop regimen impeccably. Some patients have developed adverse effects from the topical medications, such as drug allergy or toxicity reactions. Prolonged use of the steroid drops can be associated with cata-ract production or the development of steroid-induced raised intraocular pressure.

Periodic Tests and Follow-Up

You will be required to undergo certain tests including vision assessments and other measure-ments at our office before and after the procedure. Postoperative exams are scheduled every 24 to 48 hours for the first 1 to 5 days to monitor your progress after surgery. Follow-up will then be required at 1 to 2 weeks and then monthly for approximately 3 to 4 months.

If laser enhancement is required, a repeat procedure can be performed once the refraction is stable, which is usually after 6 months.

Financial Responsibility

There will be a charge for each eye depending on your candidacy for conventional treatment or customized treatment. This is the sole responsibility of the patient and must be paid in full prior to the surgery. Retreatments/enhancement surgery(s) are included in the fees for each eye for a time frame of 18 months postoperatively.

Alternate Treatment

You are free to decide not to have this operation. If you decide not to have this procedure for the correction of nearsightedness (myopia), farsightedness (hyperopia), and/or astigmatism, there are other methods of restoring vision without excimer laser surgery, including but not limited to eyeglasses, contact lenses, or other refractive surgeries depending on your ocular health.

5. Preoperative Instructions

- *Do not* wear your contact lenses prior to your surgery. Soft contact lenses must be out for 1 week and hard contact lenses must be out for 2 weeks prior to your surgery.

- You are advised to take 500 mg of vitamin C twice a day for 1 week before surgery.

- Pick up one or 2 boxes of preservative-free artificial tears (Bion [Alcon Laboratories, Fort Worth, TX] or Thera Tears [Advanced Vision Research, Ann Arbor, MI]).

- Normal activities and meals *are recommended* (breakfast and lunch) on the day of surgery. Please have something to eat and drink if/when you take the Tylenol 3 (Janssen, Raritan, NJ).

- A responsible adult *must accompany you to your residence,* even if you are traveling by taxi. You should not travel by public transportation for the remainder of the day.

- It is recommended that you do a lid wash and warm compresses for 5 minutes the night before surgery and a warm compress for 5 minutes the morning of surgery.

- *Do not* use perfume, cologne, or aftershave on the day of surgery. These products affect the laser.

- *Do not* wear any make-up. This includes powder foundation, pressed/compact powder, or blusher. You may resume the use of make-up 1 week after your surgery.

- If you are having PRK surgery on both eyes, we recommend taking 7 to 10 days off of work for recovery.

- If you are having epi-LASIK surgery on both eyes, we recommend taking 4 to 6 days off of work for recovery.

- *You may not be able to drive for 7 to 10 days.* Please make arrangements for a driver for your surgery day and your postoperative appointments.

- On the day of surgery, you will be at the surgery center for approximately 1.5 to 2 hours.

6. Postoperative Instructions

Following your surgery, do the following:

- For the first *48 hours,* use *preservative-free artificial tears* at least hourly or more often as needed while awake.

- The eye remains numb from the anesthetic drops for about 30 to 60 minutes after surgery.

- As the anesthetic drops wear off after surgery, it is normal to experience itching, burning, and watery eyes. Do not assume the watering of your eye means it is well lubricated.

- Apply a cold compress gently to the lids with the eyes closed 4 or more times per day for 48 hours following surgery.

- Limit your activities to allow for more rapid healing; you may feel most comfortable with your eyes closed.

- Avoid alcohol following surgery; sedatives and pain medication may have adverse side effects if used in combination with alcohol.

During the first week of recovery, do the following:

- Continue to keep eyes well lubricated with Refresh Tears (Allergan, Irvine, CA) 4 to 6 times per day.

- Do not drive or operate any machinery until you meet the legal motor vehicle standards vision requirements. Legal-to-drive vision is not 20/20, and you may have to limit your driving to short trips, familiar places, and daytime only to start.

- Avoid concentrated reading, computer work or games, and watching television for at least the first 6 to 12 hours after surgery. Visually demanding activities can lead to more dryness and more discomfort.

- Be cautious not to bump your eyes when removing clothing (such as a turtleneck) over your head.

- When showering or bathing, avoid getting soap in your eyes. When washing or drying your face, pat around the eyes with the facecloth or towel, and be careful not to rub your eyes.

- Avoid swimming, hot tubs, saunas, Jacuzzis, water sports, and smoky and dusty environments for 1 to 2 weeks following surgery. Regular exercise is safe; however, you may wish to wait until the bandage contact lens is removed after 4 or 5 days. Using a sweatband can help to avoid perspiration in the eyes, which can lead to irritation.

- If your eyes feel uncomfortable, it is usually an indication that you need to rest your eyes by keeping them closed for a period of time.

- Use a gentle cold compress, ice pack, or warm compress over closed eyelids for additional comfort as needed.

How to use your eye drops:

- Pred Minims (Chauvin, Surrey, UK)—preservative-free steroid eye drops that provide relief from redness, irritation, and discomfort by reducing ocular inflammation.

- FML (Allergan)—a steroid eye drop that provides relief from redness, irritation, and discomfort by reducing ocular inflammation. These drops will be started when the Pred Minims are discontinued.

- Zymar (Allergan)—an antibiotic eye drop to guard against infection.

- Acular LS (Allergan)—an anti-inflammatory to reduce the amount of inflammation.

- Tetracaine—a preservative-free freezing eye drop that will provide immediate relief when the other eye drops and oral medication fail to improve your level of comfort. These are intended to be used sparingly as overuse can delay healing.

- Preservative-free artificial tears—nonmedicated eye drops used every 30 to 60 minutes while the bandage contact lens is in place.

- Artificial tears—nonmedicated eye drops used after the bandage contact lens is removed. Artificial tears work effectively to lubricate the eyes and to keep the eyes comfortable and may reduce excessive watering. Use artificial tears up to 6 or 8 times daily as needed.

- Tylenol 3—oral medication containing codeine, which is provided for pain management if needed. Take 1 or 2 tablets as needed every 4 to 6 hours. Consult with the surgery center or with a pharmacist before combining with other prescription or non-prescription pain medications.

If the bandage contact lens falls out of your eye(s), do not re-insert the used contact lens. If you are comfortable handling contact lenses, you can re-insert the new lens provided in your medication kit. Call the office at the number provided if you need additional assistance.

7. **Frequently Asked Questions:**

- What is CustomVue Wavefront laser vision correction?

  ○ The Visx S4 IR excimer laser can use information from the Wavescan analyzer to create a highly accurate unique laser correction pattern that will correct both the standard prescription and the individual aberrations that are specific to your eye. This wavefront correction is the most advanced laser vision correction available.

- How do I decide between Advanced CustomVue Epi-LASIK and Advanced CustomVue PRK?

  ○ With epi-LASIK, visual recovery should be somewhat faster than with PRK. The long-term results are equally good with either treatment. Some people might only qualify for PRK.

  ○ No-flap treatments, such as epi-LASIK and PRK, may be safer than flap procedures such as LASIK. With LASIK, it is more complex to create the flap and the flap could be damaged or shifted even years later as a result of an eye injury. Common sense and proper use of safety glasses can prevent many eye injuries. If you have a high-risk occupation, sport, or hobby, then epi-LASIK and PRK may be a better choice for you.

- What are the risks?

  ○ With either treatment, the main risks are corneal haze or infection, which in most cases can be treated. With either treatment, the eyes may be drier and you may experience an increase in glare or halos at night. Some people may need to use an ointment at bedtime if they experience sticking eyelids or sore eyes in the morning.

  ○ For epi-LASIK, there is a small chance of corneal irregularities occurring at the time of surgery that may require additional treatment. For most people, these side effects will improve over time but in some cases, it can be permanent. You will be asked to view an informational DVD and read consent forms prior to surgery. Any factors that might increase your chances of experiencing a permanent side effect, such as dry eye, will be discussed.

- What should I expect on the day of surgery?

  ○ It is important to eat your usual meals on the day of your treatment and avoid the use of make-up, perfumes, after shave, or any other scented products. When you arrive at the center, a staff member will go over some important instructions with you, including what drops to use after surgery. Any questions you may have will be answered by a staff member.

  ○ You may wish to take a mild sedative. You will be introduced to the staff in the laser suite and positioned in the laser chair. Staff will talk you through the treatment so you will know what to expect. Freezing drops are used to numb the eye surface, and you will feel some sensations on the lids from the lid holder.

  ○ After your treatment, you will be asked to rest for a few minutes in the recovery area. You will need transportation to and from the center on the day of surgery. You will likely wish to rest for the remainder of the day following your laser vision correction treatment.

- Will it hurt?

  ○ With any laser vision correction, there will be some sensations on the lids during surgery. Most people feel a tugging sensation with blinking, but do not experience discomfort on the eye due to the use of freezing drops. With Advanced CustomVue Epi-LASIK, there will be 30 seconds of pressure during the epithelial removal at which time the vision will dim or black out and you may experience a mild aching sensation that resolves at the end of this short step. Advanced CustomVue Epi-LASIK and PRK patients will have some stinging, burning, foreign-body sensation, and light sensitivity following the treatment, which may last for 3 to 5 days until the bandage contact lens is removed. Some patients will take a mild pain medication in the first few days as the eye is healing. Sometimes, the eyes feel sticky or are difficult to open after sleeping. These sensations can last for a few days to a few weeks or months following surgery. In rare cases, it can be permanent and can require ongoing use of ointment at bedtime.

- When can I go back to my regular activities?

  ○ After Advanced CustomVue Epi-LASIK (Abbott Medical Optics, Abbott Park, IL), you may be able to go back to regular activities, including driving, in 5 to 7 days and your vision will continue to improve for several days to weeks after the procedure. Following Advanced CustomVue PRK, you will be able to return to driving and other activities in about 7 to

10 days. For both PRK and epi-LASIK, the vision may not be sharp and some patients might notice doubling and fluctuations of vision for up to 3 or 4 weeks or in some cases, 1 to 3 months. A small percentage of patients will need an enhancement for best vision. With either treatment, it may take longer for the night vision to improve and, therefore, you may wish to avoid night driving for days to weeks following laser vision correction.

- How long will I be on drops after surgery?

  ○ Antibiotic drops and anti-inflammatory drops will be used for a few days following surgery. A mild steroid drop is usually recommended on a tapering schedule for about 4 months. Artificial tears or ointment at bedtime may be needed indefinitely.

- How much does it cost?

  ○ The cost for Advanced CustomVue   Epi-LASIK and Advanced CustomVue PRK (Abbott Medical Optics) is $1850 per eye. This price includes the evaluation, testing, and all post-treatment care including retreatments for up to 18 months, if required. *Full payment is due on the day of surgery. We accept Visa, MasterCard, or certified check as payments.

8. Blepharitis Handout

Blepharitis: What is it?

Blepharitis is a common inflammation of the eyelids. It is a chronic condition that cannot be cured and may need ongoing treatment. It may be asymptomatic or can cause irritation, burning, and redness of the lids, or red eye.

People with dandruff, oily skin, or dry eyes are more frequently affected. Blepharitis can start in children or adults and can continue throughout life as a chronic condition.

Each person has bacteria on the surface of his or her skin and most will never be bothered by it. These bacteria tend to live at the base of the eyelashes on certain individuals. Bacteria play a role in overactive oil glands similar to what happens with acne. Irritation may result from the overactive oil glands causing scales and particles to form along the lashes and eyelid margins.

The effects of blepharitis are different for each person. Some people have minor irritation and itching from the scales or bacteria but others may have redness and/or a burning sensation. An allergic response to the scales or bacteria that surround them may develop.

The oils produced by the glands in the lids are important in producing good-quality tears.

People with blepharitis can have poor tear quality, which leads to dry eyes. Often, other conditions like allergies and contact lens wear may contribute to discomfort.

Treatment: Caring for Blepharitis

Blepharitis cannot be cured. It is possible to control the condition by following the instructions below:

- *Warm compresses:* at least 2 times a day (morning and evening), place a warm, moist washcloth over closed eyelids for 3 to 5 minutes. It may be necessary to remoisten it with warm water as it cools down.

  ○ This will be helpful to soften and loosen scales and other particles on the eyelids. The heat helps thin out oil secretions. Warm compresses help to prevent the development of a stye, which is an inflamed lump within an eyelid oil gland. *Never use a heating pad or microwave due to risk of burn.*

- If recommended, gently clean the base of the eyelashes with lid shampoo or dilute baby shampoo once per day.

- Avoid waterproof make-up and gently remove all make-up every night with a water-based product.

- If your doctor has prescribed an antibiotic ointment, apply a small amount at the base of the lashes using a cotton swab or fingertip at bedtime.
- *Artificial tears* may be helpful to relieve dry eye symptoms. These eye drops are available without a prescription and can be used up to 6 times per day.

If the blepharitis is not able to be controlled by the above measures, it may be necessary to add one or all of the following medications:

- Oral antibiotics will be helpful at decreasing bacterial content of the eyelids. In severe cases, it may be necessary for long-term use of tetracycline. This medication is taken orally and is routinely used by patients with a skin condition called rosacea.
- Treatment of coexisting eye conditions, such as allergies, dry eyes, or contact lens overwear, may also be needed. Treatment of facial skin problems, such as rosacea or seborrheic dermatitis, might also be recommended.

Remember: To control blepharitis, it is necessary to apply warm compresses as described twice daily and remember that medications alone are not adequate.

Glossary

aberrations: Variations in the optics of the eye measured as the difference between the theoretic ideal optical system and the measured deviation of light.

aberrometer: A device that uses infrared light to measure aberrations; used in wavefront analysis and treatments.

ablation: The process of removing corneal tissue with the excimer laser.

Airy disc: The bright central light formed by the diffraction pattern of light emitted from a point source.

aliasing: When the spatial frequency of a pattern exceeds the neural limit of retinal perception, a lower frequency pattern will be perceived.

amblyopia: Reduced vision as a result of developmental issues that limit the ability of the eye to see 20/20. A common description of amblyopia is "lazy eye."

ASA: Advanced surface ablation. An acronym used to describe the combination of wavefront treatment and surface no-flap techniques.

AST: Advanced surface treatment. An acronym used to describe the combination of wavefront treatment and surface no-flap techniques.

astigmatism: An optical condition that can result in the need for glasses. Astigmatism usually results from a cornea that is not perfectly spherical but shaped more like a football. Astigmatism is sometimes due to variations in the lens of the eye.

blepharitis: A condition related to rosacea that causes plugging of the oil glands along the eyelid margin that causes irritation, dry eye, and redness.

co-management: An arrangement between 2 qualified eye care providers in which the care of a patient is shared.

conjunctiva: The outer clear membrane that covers the white part of the eye (sclera).

consent form: The legal document that discusses the possible risks of surgery. Signing this document means you have read and understood the information on the consent form.

Anderson Penno EE. *Surface Ablation:*
Techniques for Optimum Results (pp 155-159).
© 2013 SLACK Incorporated.

corneal cross-linking: The use of riboflavin as a photosensitizer in combination with ultraviolet A to create covalent bonds between collagen fibrils.

corneal dystrophy: Conditions that can cause warpage, thinning, or other corneal changes. Corneal dystrophies, including keratoconus and pellucid, are usually hereditary.

corneal mapping: Corneal maps to display topographic and thickness information.

cycloplegia: The use of medicated drops to dilate (widen) the pupil. These drops also temporarily paralyze the focusing muscles of the eye.

cycloplegic refraction: Also called a wet refraction, which is a measurement for corrective lenses that is done after drops are instilled to relax the focusing muscles.

cyclotorsion: Rotation of the eye that can occur when lying on your back.

dilation: A synonym for cycloplegia.

diopter: An optical unit of measurement used to note the power of corrective lenses.

dry refraction: Also called a manifest refraction, which is a measurement for corrective lenses that is done without drops.

epi-LASIK: A newer type of surface no-flap laser vision correction that uses a device called an epikeratome to remove the outer surface epithelium of the cornea.

epikeratome: A device with an oscillating separator used to prepare the surface of the eye for the laser application during epi-LASIK.

excimer: Argon/fluoride laser with wavelength of 193 nanometers used for vision correction.

eye tracker: A device that moves the location of the laser application to adjust for small eye movements and keep the laser aligned throughout treatment.

farsighted: The common name for hyperopia, which means that the eye must exert focal power to see clearly even at distance.

femtosecond: An ultrafast laser used to create the corneal flap for intra-LASIK.

forme fruste: A corneal dystrophy that is not causing any vision changes; usually found by corneal mapping in people without vision problems.

glaucoma: Increased pressure inside the eye and/or damage to the optic nerve resulting in reduced peripheral vision. A variety of conditions can result in glaucoma.

higher-order aberrations: Optical variations that are more complex than simple nearsightedness, farsightedness, and astigmatism. These aberrations are treated during wavefront laser vision correction surgeries.

hyperopia: Also called farsightedness, which describes an eye that must exert focal power even to see clearly at the distance.

hysteresis: The measurement of the force-in corneal deflection generated by an air jet and the force-out corneal deflection in order to measure the corneal dampening properties which is described as the corneal resistance factor.

ICL: Implantable contact lenses (also called phakic IOL) used for nonlaser vision correction surgery.

INTACS: Intrastromal corneal ring segments. Crescent polymer plastic corneal inserts used in treatment of myopia, astigmatism, and keratoconus.

intra-LASIK: A procedure in which a corneal flap is created with the femtosecond laser used in combination with the excimer laser for laser vision correction.

intraocular: Inside the eye.

IOL: Intraocular lens implant used for cataract surgery and for clear lensectomy (refractive lensectomy), which is a nonlaser vision correction option.

iridotomy: Small holes made in the iris to provide alternative fluid circulation within the eye. Iridotomies may be done for narrow-angle glaucoma or to prepare the eye for phakic-IOL implantation.

iris recognition: The use of iris landmarks unique to every individual used to achieve a rotational adjustment during wavefront laser treatments that enhances accuracy.

KASA: Keratome-assisted surface ablation. An acronym to describe epi-LASIK.

keratoconus: A hereditary corneal dystrophy that in severe cases can lead to corneal irregularities.

keratometry: Measurements of the corneal curvature.

LASIK: Laser-assisted in situ keratomileusis. A surgery that involves creating a corneal flap with a microkeratome device for laser vision correction.

macula: The center part of the retina that is responsible for sharp central acuity. The macula is affected in age-related macular degeneration.

manifest: The term used to describe the measurement of the eye's corrective error that is done without the use of drops. This is sometimes called a dry refraction.

microkeratome: Device used to create the corneal flap during LASIK surgery.

monovision: Term used to describe correcting one eye for distance and leaving the other eye nearsighted for reading.

myopia: Technical name for nearsighted, which means that even when the eye is completely relaxed the focal point is closer than infinity.

OCT: Optical coherence tomography. The use of infrared light to create tomographic images of the eye. Routinely used for corneal, retinal, and optic nerve imaging.

opaque bubble layer: A temporary whitening of the cornea that can occur during intra-LASIK surgery.

ophthalmologist: A medical doctor (MD) with a subspecialty in eyes and eye surgery.

optometrist: A doctor of optometry (OD) who is trained in nonsurgical care of the eye.

pachymetry: Corneal thickness.

pellucid marginal dystrophy: A hereditary condition that in severe cases can cause irregularities of the cornea.

photophobia: Light sensitivity that can result from many conditions.

presbyopia: The age-related loss of focusing ability that results in the need for reading glasses, bifocals, or progressive lenses sometime after the age of 40.

PRK: Photorefractive keratectomy. The original no-flap surface laser vision correction technique introduced in North America over 20 years ago in which the surface corneal epithelial cells are removed using a manual method.

progression: The natural increase in nearsightedness in youth and young adults.

progressive: Also called a lineless bifocal; a lens with a progressively changing prescription from distance at the top, to reading or close correction at the bottom.

PTK: Phototheraputic keratectomy. The use of an excimer laser in the smoothing of corneal irregularities.

ptosis: A drooping of the upper lid that can be caused by a variety of conditions.

refraction: The measurement of the need for corrective lenses.

refractive surgery: Surgeries that reduce or eliminate the need for glasses or contact lenses; also called laser vision correction if the excimer laser is used.

regression: A healing response after laser vision correction that shifts the eye back toward the original correction.

SBK: Sub-Bowman's keratomileusis or keratectomy. A newer LASIK technique that involves creating a very thin corneal flap during LASIK surgery.

standard ablation: A term generally used to indicate that spherical and astigmatic ablation patterns are in use to differentiate it from wavefront algorithms.

strabismus: Also known as "squint" or "lazy eye"; refers to an imbalance in the muscles surrounding the eye that can result in a crossed or turned eye.

technicians: Staff who assist ophthalmologists and optometrists with vision measurements and other assessments of the eye, as well as patient counseling in some cases. Technicians are often certified by the Joint Commission on Allied Health Personnel in Ophthalmology (JCAHPO).

topography: Corneal mapping that measures the surface topography.

toric: Astigmatic. Some lenses are toric, which means they include a correction for astigmatism.

vitreous: The gel-like substance that fills the back of the eye in front of the retina but behind the lens inside the eye.

wavefront: Methods that involve the measurement of light waves exiting the eye to create a map of higher-order aberrations.

wavefront-guided: The use of wavefront maps to generate individualized treatment plans to reduce higher order aberrations.

wavefront-optimized: The use of wavefront theory to create aspheric laser ablation patterns.

Financial Disclosures

Dr. David P. Chan has not disclosed any relevant financial relationships.

Dr. Richard J. Duffey has no financial or proprietary interest in the materials presented herein.

Dr. Daniel S. Durrie receives research support from, is a consultant and clinical investigator for, and travels for Abbott Medical Optics, Alcon, and NexisVision; is on the board for Alcon and NexisVision; participates in manuscript preparation for Abbott Medical Optics and Alcon; receives lecture fees from NexisVision; and is a stock holder of Alcon and NexisVision.

Dr. Howard V. Gimbel has no financial or proprietary interest in the materials presented herein.

Dr. Harilaos Ginis has several patents in the field of mechanical epikeratomes and has served as a consultant for CIBA Vision and Norwood Eyecare for the design and development of such devices.

Dr. Maria Kalyvianaki has no financial or proprietary interest in the materials presented herein.

Dr. Alejandro Lichtinger has no financial or proprietary interest in the materials presented herein.

Dr. Ioannis Pallikaris has not disclosed any relevant financial relationships.

Dr. Theodore A. Pasquali has no financial or proprietary interest in the materials presented herein.

Dr. Ellen E. Anderson Penno has no financial or proprietary interest in the materials presented herein.

Dr. J. Bradley Randleman has no financial or proprietary interest in the materials presented herein.

Dr. David S. Rootman has no financial or proprietary interest in the materials presented herein.

Dr. Rupa D. Shah has no financial or proprietary interest in the materials presented herein.

Index